Nursing Resources for nursing instructors:

NCLEX, critical thinking, worksheets, & more with answers included.

By Deborah Wirwicz BSN, MSNED

ABDOMINAL SYSTEM 1

1. Define the following

Glycogenolysis	
glycogenesis	
Glyconeogenesis	

2. Give a brief explanation of the liver's relationship in the following.

Fats	
Proteins	
Bilirubin	
Hormones	
Vitamins	
Clotting	

3. What is cirrhosis?

4. List two causes of cirrhosis.

    a.
    b.

5. Explain what is encephalopathy and its relationship to liver failure.

ACID-BASE BALANCE 1

1. Lists three types of patients that are at risk for an acid-base imbalance.
   a.
   b.
   c.

2. What is the role of pH in acid-base balance?

3. How is the pH measured?

4. Explain why arterial blood must be used instead of venous blood when assessing the acid-base status.

5. Define the following and their values.

pH	
PaCO2	
PaO2	
HCO3	
SaO2	
Base Excess (BE)	

6. What is a chemical buffer system?

7. What is meant by compensation?

8. Explain the role of the lungs and the kidneys in maintaining acid-base imbalance.

ALLERGY 1

1. What symptoms may be observed in common seasonal allergies?

2. Briefly explain why allergies affect some people while other people are unaffected.

3. What is it called when someone has a lethal allergic reaction?

4. Is contact dermatitis an allergy? Explain your response.

5. Describe symptoms that may present in contact dermatitis.

6. Is asthma considered an allergy? Explain your response.

7. Describe symptoms that may present in asthma.

ASSESSMENT 1

1. Match the following to its correct definition.

Topic	definition
1. Inspection	a. Therapeutic touch of the human body to obtain information
2. Palpitation	b. Hitting an object against another resulting in vibrations to elicit sounds
3. Percussion	c. Use of vision and sense of smell to gather data

   1. _____ 2. _____ 3. _____

2. What is the purpose of a nursing assessment?

3. What is the difference between an initial nursing assessment and a shift assessment?

4. Which of the assessment skills in the box above would be used to assess a skin rash?

5. Which of the assessment skills in the box above would be used to assess pulses?

6. Which of the assessment skills in the box above would be used to assess a distended abdomen?

7. Which of the assessment skills in the box above would be used to assess a pressure ulcer?

8. What is auscultation?

9. Which organ would you use the diaphragm and the bell of your stethoscope to auscultate?

10. Which skill would be first when assessing respirations, auscultation, or inspection?

11. Explain a problem that may occur when palpating a pulse.

12. Which skills may be involved to assess the capillary refill.

BASIC NURSING KNOWLEDGE 1

1. List the areas that intramuscular injections may be administered.

2. List the areas that a subcutaneous injection may be administered.

3. List the veins that an intravenous infusion catheter may be inserted. List which veins you would access first.

4. What is a saline lock?
   _____
   _____.

5. What is a continuous infusion?
   _____
   _____.

6. What does incompatibility refer to when discussing intravenous infusions?
   _____
   _____.

7. What is a bolus?
   _____
   _____.

8. When would a bolus be used?
   _____
   _____.

BIOTERRORISM RESEARCH PROJECT

Research your chosen community. Collect data on actual and potential bioterrorism situations. Put together a power point, spread sheet, or report on the collected data.

List (in each discovered situation) the following:

1. First responders at local level. who are the first responders? What plan do they implement? Who takes charge? What is a command center and why would one be needed? What resources would be available?

2. First responders at the state level. Who are the first responders? How do they play a role in an event that occurs at the local level? What plan do they implement? Who takes charges? What resources would be available?

3. First responders at the national level. Who are the first responders? How do they play a role in the event that occurs at the local and state level? What plan do they implement? Who takes charge? What resources would be available?

4. First responders at the international level. What type of situations could occur at the international level? Is there an organization that is specific to international crisis? What resources would be available and where would they originate?

BLOOD TRANSFUSION WORKSHEET

1.	Does not have antigens	A.
2.	Type A + may receive these blood types	B.
3.	Type B+ may receive these blood types	C.
4.	Type AB+ may receive these blood types	D.
5.	Type AB- may receive these blood types	E.
6.	Type O + may receive these blood types	F.
7.	Type O – may receive these blood types	G.
8.	Is considered the universal donor	H.
9.	Is considered the universal recipient	I.
10.	Type A – may receive these blood types	J.
11.	Type B- may receive these blood types	K.

1. List the four blood types: _____, _____, _____, _____.

Match the following to the appropriate response

What is the maximum duration red blood cells can be transfused? _____ _____.
A. What is the duration fresh frozen plasma can be transfused? _____ _____.
B. What is the duration platelets can be transfused? _____.

CARDIAC 1

1. Define the following and list their role in caring for a cardiac patient

Echocardiogram	
Stress test	
Troponin	
Myoglobin	
Cholesterol	
HDL	
LDL	
Triglycerides	

2. Define the difference between the following

ANGINA	MYOCARDIAL INFARCTION

3. What is heart failure?

CARDIAC 2

1. List the difference between right ventricular and left ventricular heart failure.

Left ventricular heart failure	Right ventricle heart failure

2. Which cardiac ventricle pumps blood into the periphery?
3. Which cardiac ventricle pumps blood to the lungs?
4. When would JVD be observed?
5. When would peripheral edema be observed?
6. List the four valves of the heart.

7. Define the following

Cardiac output (CO)	
Stroke volume	

CARDIAC 3

1. List signs and symptoms a patient with congested heart failure may demonstrate.

2. List the different causes of heart failure.

Modifiable	Nonmodifiable

3. What other health care team members should be included in the heart failure patient's care and their role?

Healthcare team member	Role in the patient's care

4. Patient teaching is important. Explain what patient education, you as the nurse, would give the heart failure patient.

Education	Rationale

CARDIAC 4

1. Describe techniques for auscultating your patient's heart sounds.

2. What are considered normal heart sounds?

3. What are considered abnormal heart sounds?

4. What is a murmur?

5. List two issues that would cause a murmur.

6. Your patient is grossly obese. His weight makes it difficult to hear heart sounds. Is there anything that can be done to assist to hear the heart sounds? Explain your answer.

7. What valves make the S1 heart sound?

8. What valves make the S2 heart sound?

9. Should the nurse use the diaphragm or bell of the stethoscope to auscultate heart sounds? Explain your response.

10. Where would you auscultate the apical pulse?

11. While auscultating your patient's heart, you note the heart rhythm is irregular with a varying rate. What rhythm would you anticipate this patient to be diagnosed with? Explain your response.

12. While auscultating your patient's heart, you hear a strange rubbing sound. Since you know the heart normally makes a S1 and S2 sound, should you be concerned? Explain your response.

CARDIAC 5

1. List five symptoms a patient in heart failure may demonstrate on admission.

2. How can heart failure affect activities of daily living?

3. List three causes of heart failure.

4. List signs or symptoms of deteriorating heart failure.

5. What patient education should be discussed with a patient that has been newly diagnosed with heart failure?

6. Why is it important for the diagnosed cardiac patient to follow a low sodium diet?

7. What is the purpose of obtaining a daily weight in the patient with a history of heart failure?

CARDIAC 6

Match the following

Cardiac drug	
1. Ace inhibitor	a. Lowers blood pressure and decreases heart rate
2. Angiotensin receptor blocker (ARB)	b. Rids the body of excess fluid. Decreases swelling.
3. Beta blocker	c. Alters hormones that may cause damage to the heart
4. diuretic	d. lowers blood pressure and decreases the work load of the heart
5. aldosterone antagonist	e. lowers heart rate. Helps the heart pump more efficiently
6. antiarrhythmic	f. lowers blood pressure and decreases the work load of the heart

1. _____ 2. _____ 3. _____ 4. _____ 5. _____ 6. _____

2. Why should patients on cardiac medications be made aware of over-the-counter (OTC) drug interaction?

3. Explain the relationship between stress and heart failure.

4. Explain how smoking affects the heart.

5. What is an echocardiogram?

6. What information can be obtained from an echocardiogram?

7. What is an ejection fraction?

8. What is a normal ejection fraction?

9. What is an electrocardiogram?

10. What does idiopathic mean?

CHARTING SCAVENGER HUNT

List where you would chart or find the following in an electronic medical record.

1. Allergies
2. Activity level
3. To enter home medications
4. Modify allergies
5. R.N. assessment
6. Primary diagnosis
7. Vaccination history
8. Tobacco, alcohol, or substance usage
9. Advance directive
10. Weight and height
11. Intake and output with 24-hour total
12. Vital signs
13. Pain assessment
14. Neurological assessment
15. Heart murmurs
16. Oxygen usage
17. Date indwelling urinary catheter was inserted
18. IV site
19. Fall risk

20. Laboratory results

COMMUNITY ASSIGNMENT

Assess your community. Plan a needs plan for your community. Include what resources maybe needed to achieve your plan. Be certain to add expected expenses or cost lists to get your plan up and running.

Assessment: the need of the community. Ideas can be veterans small homes, a free clinic, transportation, language instructors, or playground.

Diagnosis: what is the problem in the community that needs focus

Plan: who will implement the plan and what is the time line.

Evaluation: what evidence would demonstrate your project has met its goals?

COMMUNITY RESEARCH PROJECT

Choose one of the topics below. Research how your community addresses this issue. Meet with public agency members to obtain statistics and additional data.

1. Drugs of abuse
2. Gambling
3. Sexual addiction
4. Teenage smoking
5. Alcoholism
6. Domestic violence
7. Maternal health
8. Birth control
9. End-of-life care
10. Shelter needs

COMMUNITY WINDSHIELD SURVEY PROJECT

Gather information on your chosen community. Take pictures of your community (have someone drive while you take pictures to ensure safety) and develop a power point with all the following information:

1. geographical information

2. social availability

3. annual incomes (include median income)

4. education (at all levels)

5. employment status (occupation)

6. housing availability and costs (include prices of purchased homes and rent)

7. languages spoken

8. assistance programs (SNAP, WIC)

9. transportation (owned vehicles, buses, trains, bicycles)

10. poverty status

11. industries

12. marital statuses

13. any military affiliations (veterans, or bases)

14. how many births and deaths annually

15. religious affiliations

16. clinics, hospitals, long-term-care facilities, or assisted living residents

17. race and ethnicity

18. age and gender of population

19. deaths

There are several sites that can offer statistical data: The U.S. Census bureau (www.census.gov.), administrative records, health department and the library.

Conversion practice worksheet

1. 2 g = _____ mg

2. 1 mg = _____ mcg

3. 25,000 mcg = _____ mg

4. 3 L = _____ mL

5. 125 mcg = _____ mg

6. 275 mL = _____ L

7. 2.5 L = _____ mL

8. 3 tsp = _____ T

9. 8 oz. = _____ mL

10. ½ gallon = _____ oz.

11. 0.5 mg = _____ mcg

12. 2.65000 mg = _____ g

13. 30 oz. = _____ mL

14. 4 oz. = _____ C

15. 15 oz. = _____ T

16. 10 mL = _____ tsp

CRITICAL CARE 1

1. List examples of cardiac emergencies.

2. List those who would be needed at the bedside of a code blue and their role

3. List at least two certifications a nurse working in a critical care area, such as ER, OR, ICU, may require.

CRITICAL CARE 2

1. List when an MRI (magnetic resonance imaging) would be contraindicated.

2. What must the nurse ensure prior to taking the patient for an ordered MRI?

3. What is cardiac monitoring? List reasons it may be used.

4. What is telemetry? List when telemetry may be used.

5. What is hemodynamic monitoring? When would hemodynamic monitoring be used?

6. Define the following.

CVP	
PAP	
PAWP	
CO	

CRITICAL CARE 3

Match the type of trauma with cause of injury using the trauma key below.

Type of trauma	Cause of trauma
1.	asphyxiation
2.	Wires downed
3.	fire
4.	Motor vehicle crash (MVC)
5.	lighting
6.	toxins
7.	Ultra violet (UV) rays
8.	steam
9.	fall
10.	Gun shot wound (GSW)
11.	substances
12.	drowning
13.	assault
14.	heat
15.	radioactive
16.	Carbon monoxide/dioxide inhalation
17.	sockets

Trauma key:

Mechanical trauma

Thermal trauma

Chemical trauma

Electrical trauma

Radiant trauma

Oxygen deprivation

CRITICAL CARE 4

1. Briefly explain how acceleration-deceleration injuries occur.
2. What is a coup-contrecoup?
3. Explain the difference between the following fractures.
    a. Linear fracture
    b. Depressed fracture
    c. Basilar skull fracture
4. Why must a patient with a traumatic brain injury need a cranial nerve assessment?
5. Why must a patient with a traumatic brain injury be monitored for a cerebral spinal fluid leak?
6. What is parenchyma?

Briefly define each of the following and their location

1. Brain tissue

2. Pia matter

3. Meninges

4. Cerebrum

5. Cerebellum

6. Brain stem

DEATH AND DYING 1

1. List three people that the family of your dying patient may request to see.
   a.
   b.
   c.

2. Your patient's widow asks, "Did my husband have a lot of pain before he died?" What is your response if you were unable to make the patient completely comfortable. Explain your response.

3. Your dying patient is listed as an organ donor. What would you need to do or contact?

4. List two things you, as the nurse, can do for yourself to assist in dealing with the grief from caring for your dying patient?
   a.
   b.

5. What is comfort care?

6. What is euthanasia?

7. Is euthanasia legal? If so, list where and when is it legal (if applicable)?

8. What are the five stages of grief as per the Kubler-Ross model.

9. Does a dying patient go through the five stages of grief in order? Explain your answer.

DELEGATION & LICENSURE 1

1. List the relationship between supervision and delegation. Briefly explain each role.

2. List the five factors that must be met before a nurse may delegate a task.

3. Once a task is delegated, can that task be re-delegate? Explain your response.

4. Must all delegated tasks be supervised? Explain your response.

5. List the nursing personnel that are allowed to delegate. Explain which staff cannot delegate and the reason why.

6. Explain what should be done if you are assigned a task that you have not been trained to perform?

7. Each state determines the scope of practice of a nurse. What other limitations may be imposed and by what those limitations are imposed by.

8. Explain the differences between responsibility and accountability.

9. When a task is delegated, who is ultimately accountable to ensure the task was completed.

10. What should the nurse do if the patient-care-technician is assigned a task but fails to complete the task or explain why the task was not completed?

EAR 1

1. What is otitis media?

2. List three characteristics of an inner ear problem and give description of each.

3. List an inner ear disease and briefly describe it.

4. What is an acoustic neuroma?

5. What is a benign paroxysmal vertigo and when does it occur?

6. What safety issue may occur when a patient has an inner or middle ear infection. Explain your answer.

7. List four ototoxic medications.

26

8. What is a common physical finding in a patient with a middle ear infection?

9. What is cerumen?

EMERGENT CARE

1. Define what is triage and how may triage be used in healthcare.

2. List the classification levels of triage and an example of each.

3. List the equipment used in standard precautions.

4. In an emergent situation. a primary survey must be performed. List the ABCDE of the survey.

27

5. What is a rapid response team? List the members of the rapid response team.

ETHICS WORKSHEET 1

1. Must a child be given complete disclosure regarding their health issue or status? Explain your response.

2. A 14-year-old girl is in active labor. Can the patient make her own decisions or must her parents be contacted to give consent? Explain your response.

3. A mother and her daughter have been living on the streets. The mother is brutally stabbed. The 14-year-old daughter runs from the assailant and is hit by a bus. The girl is taken to the emergency room and pronounced brain dead. Can this patient be an organ donor? Explain the ethical dilemma involved in this case.

4. A patient is admitted with severe arthritis. The patient states, "I don't want to live with this pain any longer." Explain the difference between chronic pain and quality of life in this patient.

5. Explain the difference between a dependent patient and an independent patient.

6. An 80-year-old widow is admitted with malnutrition. Your co-worker states this patient is part of the vulnerable population. Explain what is a vulnerable population and how this patient meets those criteria?

7. You are assigned a patient who has a DNR on his chart. The patient is intubated. What is a DNR and how is this situation an ethical dilemma?

8. Define justice and explain how it plays a role in healthcare.

9. You overhear one of your coworkers say to her patient, "Dr. Purple is a quack. You should get a different doctor." Explain how this statement is slander and what repercussions can result.

10. Explain the difference between neglect and abandonment.

11. Explain how failure to document in the electronic medical record (EMR) can result in an ethical dilemma. Give an example.

ETHICS WORKSHEET 2

Match the following to its appropriate definition

1. Credentialling
2. Certification
3. Licensure
4. Autonomy
5. Supervision
6. Beneficence
7. Justice
8. Nonmaleficence
9. Unlicensed
10. Delegation
11. Competence

a. Self-determination and decision making
b. Legal authority to perform medical interventions and procedures
c. Actions for the welfare of others
d. Fairness to all
e. Qualification entitling the right to defined power
f. Assignment of a task or mission
g. Attesting to a level of achievement
h. Lacking legal authority
i. Do no harm
j. Facilitates control
k. Ability to perform efficiently

Answers:

1. _____   2. _____   3. _____   4. _____   5. _____
6. _____   7. _____   8. _____   9. _____   10. _____
11. _____

ETHICS WORKSHEET 3

1. Research a bioethics topic, such as stem cells. List the ethical pros and cons of your chosen topic. Explain which side you favor and why.

2. Define autonomy.

3. Explain how autonomy relates to nursing.

4. Explain how autonomy relates to patient choices.

5. Define disclosure.

6. Explain the legal position of a nurse regarding informed consent for a patient who may become a research candidate.

7. Define nonmaleficence.

8. Explain how non-maleficence plays a role in research or post operative care.

9. Give an example of a situation in which a nurse may advocate for the patient.

10. List the people that maybe involved in making clinical decisions for a patient. Explain how they maybe come involved in the decision-making process.

11. Explain the self-determination act when the patient is mentally incompetent.

12. Define integrity.

13. How does integrity affect the nurse when assuming the role of patient advocate?

14. Is caring a legal or professional requirement for a nurse? Explain your answer.

ETHICS WORKSHEET 4

1. Define precedence.

2. How does precedence play a role in nursing? Give an example.

3. Define competence.

4. How does healthcare ensure the nurse is competent? Give an example

5. Define assault.

6. Define battery

7. Give an example of assault.

8. Give an example of battery.

9. Give an example of false imprisonment of a patient.

10. What is defamation?

11. Define HIPAA

12. List five examples of how a nursing student can maintain HIPAA when participating in nursing clinical classes.

13. Define negligence

14. Give an example of neglect.

15. Explain the relationship between neglect and malpractice.

16. A patient's condition is terminal but the family wants everything done. To continue medical care would cause prolonged pain for the patient. Who should make the determination of ceasing further life-prolonging care if the patient is unable?

ETHICS WORKSHEET 5

1. Using one of the included ethical dilemmas, explain what YOU would do ethically as a nurse for the patient.
    a. A suicidal patient
    b. A patient refusing a blood transfusion but will die without this intervention
    c. A 13-year-old wanting an abortion
    d. A patient seeking an assisted death

2. What is a living will?

3. What is medical power of attorney? Do they have limitations? Explain your answer.

4. Choose one of the included scenarios. Explain how you would advocate for the patient if you were the assigned nurse.

a. A patient that no longer wants her life prolonged by chemotherapy
   b. A patient with a living will that states no life support has severe pneumonia
   c. A patient with malignant gallstones who doesn't want surgery
   d. A ventilated brain-dead patient who is listed as an organ donor but the family refuses

5. List members of the healthcare team and a brief description of their role.

6. Define collaboration.

7. How does collaboration with other healthcare team members play a role in the nurse-patient relationship?

8. A married couple choses to have the wife's eggs frozen. Years later, they are divorced. The wife wants the eggs destroyed. The husband wants the eggs to survive. Explain who decides reproductive rights and privileges. How does this play a role in ethical and legal issues.

9. The doctor writes an order. YOU as the nurse believes it is in error. Explain what, if anything, you can do.

10. You are assigned a patient that states, "I only use osteopathic medications and methods." Explain what osteopathic is and it will affect your care of the patient.

ETHICS WORKSHEET 6

An ethical dilemma is when a decision must be made between two choices which involve moral principles.

1. Describe a situation with a dilemma that you have encountered. This dilemma could be personal, at work, or observed.

2. Describe a situation with an **ethical** dilemma you have encountered. This dilemma could be personal, at work, or observed.

3. Explain which side you would choose and the moral principal that determined the final choice.

4. A hospital must be caution with money spending. The hospital signs a contract with a supply company that makes necessary patient care items, however; the items are cheap and of poor quality. Urinary drainage bags leak which can result in increased patient infections, falls from wet floors, and increased cost due to the need for multiple replacements. Is this an ethical dilemma? Explain your response.

5. The family of a Covid-19 patient on a ventilator in the intensive care unit is dying. The family requests the patient to receive "last rites." The nondenominal clergy is willing to give the requested service but isolation supplies (gowns, masks, and gloves) are limited. The clergy cannot go to the bedside as his use of supplies is considered non-essential. Is this an ethical dilemma? Explain your response.

EYES 1

1. List two types of macular degeneration. Give a brief description of each.

2. What are cataracts?

3. Listed below are three types of cataracts. List where each type forms.

Subcapsular	
Nuclear	
Cortical	

4. List risk factors for cataracts.

5. Your patient has a visual opacity of the left eye. What do you assess the opacity to be?

6. List two risk factors for dry macular degeneration.

The doctor has performed cataract surgery on your patient. How would you prevent the patient from rubbing the surgical eye?

EYE 2

1. Briefly explain what may be diagnosed in the patient with increased intraocular pressure.

2. What can cause increased intraocular pressure?

3. List two types of glaucoma and give a brief definition of each.

a.	
b.	

4. What is a complication of untreated glaucoma?

5. What is a Snellen chart? How is it used?

6. Define what each letter in PERRLA means.

P	
E	
R	
R	
L	
A	

FETUS 1

1. What is an alpha fetoprotein test? Include what abnormal levels indicate in your response.

2. What is an amniocentesis and when would it be considered?

3. What is the purpose of monitoring HCG (human chorionic gonadotrophin)?

4. What is the purpose of karyotyping?

5. List the risk of CVS (chorionic villus sampling).

6. When would an amniotic fluid aspiration be performed?

7. List what may compromise a vaginal delivery.

8. Explain what are Braxton Hicks contractions?

9. How does the nurse know the fetus is progressing for delivery?

10. What does it mean if the effacement is partial?

11. At what stage of labor would an epidural be offered?

12. What is an episiotomy and at what stage of labor may a mother require one?

13. At what stage of labor is the placenta expelled?

14. What is the purpose of a uterine massage?

15. What is the purpose of the APGAR score?

16. What is one of the biggest problem with a new born?

17. List interventions to prevent hypothermia of the infant.

18. When and why would the nurse need to monitor the infant's glucose levels?

FLUIDS AND ELECTROLYTES 1

1. Explain how fluids and electrolytes are distributed though out the body.

2. List three ways a patient may lose fluids.

3. List two causes of electrolyte and fluid imbalance that may occur because of therapeutic treatment.

4. List the four main electrolytes in the body.

5. What is the relationship between electrolytes and IV nutritional therapy?

6. Define the following.

topic	definition
osmosis	
diffusion	
Active transport	
filtration	

7. Explain the difference between sensible and insensible losses.

8. Explain how the kidney plays a role in the regulation of fluid and electrolytes.

9. Explain how hormones play a role in the regulation of fluid and electrolytes.

10. Explain the difference between isotonic, hypertonic, and hypotonic.

11. List the risks factors involved in fluid volume deficit. (remember injuries can play a part)

12. List the risks factors involved in fluid volume excess.

FLUID AND ELECTROLYTES 2

List the risk factors of the following electrolyte abnormalities.

1. Hyponatremia

2. Hypernatremia

3. Hypokalemia

4. Hyperkalemia

5. Hypocalcemia

6. Hypercalcemia

7. Hypomagnesia

8. Hypermagnesia

9. Hypophosphatemia

10. Hyperphosphatemia

List two risk factors or causes for each of the following conditions

1. Metabolic acidosis

2. Metabolic alkalosis

3. Respiratory acidosis

4. Respiratory alkalosis

FLUID AND ELECTROLYTES 3

1. List two ways to assess a patients hydration status.

2. Explain how fluid and electrolytes help to maintain the body's stable environment.

3. List two diseases that may affect fluid and electrolyte balances.

4. Give an example of a treatment in which the nurse must anticipate a potential fluid and electrolyte imbalance. Explain why this imbalance occurs.

5. Name two fluid compartments of the body and which electrolyte is of higher concentration.

6. List two areas of the body that contain extracellular fluid.

7. List three locations in the body with transcellular fluid.

List the locations of the following	LOCATION
Interstitial fluid	
Intravascular fluid	
Lymph fluid	
transcellular	

List if the following electrolytes are positive or negatively charged.	NEGATIVE OR POSITIVELY CHARGED
SODIUM	
POTASSIUM	
CALCIUM	
MAGNESIUM	
CHLORIDE	

FOUNDATIONS IN NURSING WORKSHEET 1

1. Define professionalism. Explain how to become a professional.

2. Define an occupation. What is the difference between an occupation and a profession?

3. What is the definition of nursing per the American Nursing Association.

4. What is meant be the art of nursing?

5. What is meant by the science of nursing?

6. What type of nursing degree can a student attain from a community college?

7. What type of nursing degree can a student attain from a university?

8. What is accreditation and how does it play a role in healthcare?

9. Why is accreditation important when applying for a nursing program?

10. What characteristics should a nurse possess? Explain your answer.

11. What is the purpose of nursing organizations?

12. Who makes up the regulatory licensing boards?

13. List the various roles a nurse may choose to work.

14. List the various types of healthcare services available in your community.

15. What is the nursing scope of practice? List the six factors in the scope of nursing.

16. Explain what the duties of a nurse means and how it differs from obligation.

17. What is the nursing process?

18. List the steps of the nursing process.

19. What is the standards of nursing practice.

FOUNDATIONS OF NURSING WORKSHEET 2

1. How should a nurse introduce himself/herself to the patient?

2. List several ways in which a nursing student or new nurse can promote or maintain patient dignity.

3. If the patient states, "I don't want a student nurse assigned to me," what should the student do?

4. Define holistic. Give an example of how a holistic problem may impact patient care.

5. How is competence determined in a health care professional?

6. What are professional boundaries? Give an example

7. What is therapeutic communication? Explain why it is important in nursing.

8. List four different types of therapeutic communication techniques. Give an example of each.

9. Explain the relationship between nursing and honesty.

10. How does truth play a role in healthcare?

11. Define culture.

12. How does culture play a role in healthcare?

13. Can social media play a role in healthcare? Explain your answer

14. Define discrimination.

15. List two examples of discrimination in healthcare.

16. Explain how professional behavior in nursing plays a role in how nurses are viewed by the public.

FOUNDATIONS OF NURSING WORKSHEET 3

1. What is a nurse?

2. How can a nurse use warm and caring communication techniques to improve patient participation in their care? Give an example.

3. How can non-verbal communication cause an issue in patient participation? Explain your answer.

4. Explain why the patient is given a patient-bill-of-rights on admission.

5. Explain the difference between rights and responsibilities.

6. How does the patient-bill-of-rights empower the patient and his/her family?

7. What is a nursing plan of care?

8. Explain the importance of the nursing plan of care. Include how collaboration plays a role.

9. Is it true, once a nurse completes the nursing program and passes the state board of nursing examination, there is no further educational requirements needed? Explain your answer.

10. Is it true, when an ethical issue arises, the nurse can take time to contemplate the situation before determining an intervention? Explain your response.

11. List ways in which to facilitate discussions when an ethical and clinical conflict occurs.

12. List ways to teach a new nurse how to become a patient advocate. Give an example of each response.

13. List examples of non-therapeutic communication phrases that can block effective communication between the nurse and the patient.

14. Explain why healthcare systems are focusing on patient safety. Give an example of a way in which the healthcare system promotes a safe environment.

15. Give an example of how a nurse can avoid non-therapeutic communication.

FOUNDATIONS OF NURSING WORKSHEET 4

1. Your patient asks you, "what is my diagnosis?" Can you, as the assigned nurse give your patient their diagnosis, prognosis, and potential treatment plan? Explain your answer.

2. Often patients and their families feel vulnerable and powerless. Their lack of knowledge of the healthcare arena, routines, and protocols makes them fearful. Why must the nurse interpret the patient and family's position and ensure other healthcare team members recognize the needs and preferences of the patient and family?

3. Explain why the nurse must maintain professional boundaries.

4. List issues of cultural diversity that may arise in healthcare.

5. How can the nurse or healthcare system ensure cultural diversity is incorporated into the patient's plan of care? Give an example

6. Explain how you, as the nurse, can facilitate coordination of the interdisciplinary team.

7. As a patient's health improves, it is often necessary to transfer the patient to an external healthcare facility. Explain how the interdisciplinary team must work together to ensure this process.

8. Explain the difference between managed care, a health maintenance organization (HMO) and a preferred provider organization (PPO).

9. Explain what the federal false claims act is and how it pertains to kick backs, false claims in billing, and self-referrals.

10. What is risk management?

11. What is the relationship between risk management and nursing?

12. What is the difference between people skills and technical skills?

13. What is quality improvement or quality assurance and how does it play a role in patient care?

FOUNDATIONS OF NURSING WORKSHEET 5

1. What is evidence-based-practice (EBP)?

2. Where did the nursing profession originally get its skills and knowledge?

3. Why is EBP important in nursing?

4. List the interdisciplinary team and their role in patient rounds.

5. What is informatics?

6. Has informatics improved healthcare? Explain your response.

7. List two new challenges informatics bring to HIPAA regulations.

8. Explain the relationship between quality improvement and EBP.

9. How can the care based on EBP be documented in the patient's plan of care as a positive performance outcome?

10. Problem-solving is a skill the nurse must learn. A problem may occur due to poor communication, culture, or patient beliefs. Give an example of situation that may occur based on the three issues listed and how you as the nurse would problem solve the situation.

G.I. SYSTEM 1

1. Your patient has been diagnosed with a G.I. Bleed. The stool is black, and tarry. Based on your findings, is this an upper G.I. bleed or a lower G.I. Bleed? Explain your rationale.

2. What information would you want to gather from the GI bleed patient?

Information	Rationale

3. List five interventions that would be appropriate for a patient with an upper G.I. bleed.

Interventions	Rationale

G.I. SYSTEM 2

1. A patient admitted status post (S/P) motor vehicle crash (MVC). The patient's car was T-boned. From the force, the patient's car then spun and hit a light pole. The patient is complaining of left upper quad pain. Lists the possible causes of this patient's pain.

2. What tests might be appropriate for this patient? Include your rationale for each test.

Test	rationale

3. What past medical history might you want to include in the patient's medical record?

Information	Rationale

GI SYSTEM 3

1. Your patient with a nasogastric tube is complaining of nausea. What interventions will you provide?

Interventions	Rationale

2. The patient fell off a high ladder and is diagnosed with a spinal injury. The doctor orders the patient to be logrolled. What is logrolled and why is it ordered?

3. The doctor orders your patient to be in the supine position. The patient begins to complain that the medication has made him nauseated. What interventions will you provide? Explain your rationale.

Intervention	Rationale

4. The pulse oximetry alarm on the contracted patient with a continuous tube feeding is sounding. You enter the room and see the patient's mouth is full of tube feeding. List your actions based on priority.

GI SYSTEM 4

Match the following. Draw an arrow from the GI subject to the correct definition.

GI subject	Definition
1. colectomy	a. blocked colon
2. total colectomy	b. inflammation of the bowel resulting in sores
3. partial colectomy	c. inflammation of the bowels
4. hemicolectomy	d. removal of the left or right colon
5. proctocolectomy	e. entire colon and rectum removed
6. bowel obstruction	f. Surgical removal of the colon or a section removed
7. Crohn's disease	g. Entire colon removed
8. Ulcerative colitis	h. part of colon removed

1. What is a P.E.G.?

2. What is a nasogastric tube (NGT) and why is it ordered?

3. Can a patient receive medications and tube feeding via a nasogastric tube?

4. How is nasogastric tube placement initially confirmed?

5. Why is an X-ray required to confirm the placement of a nasogastric tube?

6. A patient with an NGT is coughing a lot. What would be the nurse's concern?

7. The patient who has been receiving a continuous tube feeding via a NGT has a distended abdomen. What would you assess?

HEALTH AND WELLNESS

1. List at minimal six aspects of health and wellness.
   _____
   _____
   _____.

2. List two ways a patient's health can be affected.
   _____
   _____.

3. List three of each of the following factors that affect health.

Modifiable	Non-modifiable

4. List ways in which a patient may meet a desired outcome.
   _____
   _____.

5. Explain what is the illness to wellness continuum.
   _____
   _____
   _____.

6. Define illness.
   _____
   _____.

7. List obstacles that may prevent a patient from complying with necessary health changes or lifestyle changes.
   _____
   _____
   _____
   _____.

HORMONE 1

1. List the signs and symptoms of Cushing's syndrome and Cushing's disease. List the differences as well as similar signs and symptoms.

Health issue	Signs/symptoms	Similar signs	Different signs
Cushing's syndrome			
Cushing's disease			

2. The patient says he is between jobs and can't afford the steroid medication. He has one week's worth of medication remaining. He asks you if he can just stop or does he need to keep taking the steroid medication. How would you respond? Explain your rationale.

3. List the differences between the two hormones below.

Hormone	Benefits	Side effects
Glucocorticoid		
Mineralocorticoid		

INFANT 1

1. When assessing the pulse of the newborn infant, list the sites and expected heart rate.

2. Would you expect to hear infant bowel sounds immediately after birth? Explain your response.

3. What is the purpose of eye prophylaxis?

4. What is the purpose of phytonadione?

5. What may cause jaundice in an infant?

6. What are Mongolian spots?

7. What are typical assessment factors in an infant examination?

8. What are the characteristics of fetal alcohol syndrome?

9. When should the infant have their first stool?

10. What are the characteristics of an infant born to a substance addicted mother?

11. Briefly explain how a blood sample is obtained from an infant.

12. What is the purpose of an incubator?

13. Why are caps placed on the infant's head?

14. What considerations should be taken when bathing the infant?

INFECTION WORKSHEET

Match the following:

		Match letter with number
A. Abscess	1. Cell death	a.
B. Exudate	2. A vulnerability	b.
C. Transudate	3. Accumulation of purulent material	c.
D. Inflammation	4. Fluid that seeps from blood vessels or organs	d.
E. Necrosis	5. Intervention to reduce risk of transmission	e.
F. Nosocomial	6. Fluids that pass through a membrane	f.
G. Purulent	7. Discharge	g.
H. Vector	8. A reaction to tissue	h.
I. Susceptibility	9. Transmits a pathogen	i.
J. Standard precautions	10. hospital acquired	j.

Match the precaution		
A. airborne	1. MRSA, VRE, ESBL, C-diff, Conjunctivitis, RSV, impetigo, lice, and scabies	a.
B. Droplet	Chickenpox, measles, tuberculosis	b.
C. Contact	Whooping cough, pneumonia, diphtheria, adenovirus, meningococcal, mumps, and scarlet fever	c.

INTEGUMENTARY SYSTEM 1

1. Define Exudate: _____.

2. Define transudate: _____.

3. Explain the difference between a bedsore and a pressure ulcer.
   _____
   _____
   _____
   _____.

4. List the anticipated duration of healing in the following pressure-ulcers stages.

Stage 1	
Stage 2	
Stage 3	
Stage 4	

5. Explain how a pressure ulcer is measured?

6. List what should be assessed each time a dressing is changed.

7. What is eschar and how is it is treated?

8. What color is granulation tissue?

9. You are precepting. You must explain to the student nurse what tunneling means. Explain what tunneling means how is it measured?

INTEGUMENTARY SYSTEM 2

1. Explain epidermis and why it's important.

2. Explain the health benefits of darker skin.

3. What are Merkel cells?

4. What is the primary function of skin?

5. Cana skin be a delivery system for medication? Explain your response.

6. Define endogenous and its relationship with vitamin D.

7. List potential causes of the following skin colors.

Jaundice	
Delayed wound healing	
Cyanosis	
Pallor	

8. Define the following.
   Psoriasis: _____.
   Pruritis: _____.
   Ecchymosis: _____.

9. List what changes in the skin that should be assessed.
_____
_____
_____
_____.

INTEGUMENTARY SYSTEM 3

1. What is an angioma?
2. List what is petechiae and its cause.
3. What is the difference between turgor and texture of the skin?
4. Your surgical patient has a history of keloids. What is a keloid?
5. Your patient loves to lie in the sun. On cloudy days, the patient uses a tanning bed. Could this practice cause problems with the skin? Explain your answer.
6. Some medications can potentiate the suns effects on the skin. Explain what this means and what, if anything, can be done.
7. What is contact dermatitis?
8. Explain why the following are important when assessing a mole.

Asymmetry	
Border irregularity	
Color change	
Diameter of 6 mm or larger	
Evolving	

9. What is a melanoma?
10. What is the most common cause of skin cancer?

Laboratory results

Print a copy of the laboratory form on the following page. Record the patients laboratory results. Note in the comment section what is the cause of an abnormal laboratory result.

Include what laboratory results should be monitored for the patient and the rationale why. Example: The patient's potassium level is 3.2. The patient is on digoxin and Lasix. A low potassium level will cause digoxin toxicity if the Lasix is administered. This can put your patient into a health threatening situation. The doctor would need to be notified. You would anticipate the doctor placing orders to replace the potassium. Recheck laboratory tests to ensure the potassium level is adequate to administer the digoxin and the Lasix.

	TEST			COMMENTS
	WBC			
	RBC			
	HGB			
	HCT			
	MVC			
	MCH			
	NEUTROPHILS			
	BANDS			
	LYMPHOCYTES			
	MONOCYTES			
	EOSINOPHILS			
	BASOPHILS			
	PLATELETS			
	PT			
	PTT			
	INR			
	NA (SODIUM)			
	K (POTASSIUM)			
	CHLORIDE			
	CO2			
	GLUCOSE			
	BUN			
	PHOSPHATE			
	MAGNESIUM			
	TBILIRUBIN			

	CHOLESTEROL			
	TRIGYLCERIDES			
	ALBUMIN			
	TOTAL PROTEIN			
	CPK			
	LDH			
	SGOT (AST)			
	SGPT (ALT)			
	AMYLASE			
	SERUM OSMOLARITY			
	CORTISOL			
	TSH			
	T3			
	T4			

LAW WORKSHEET 1

1. Your patient's family member was pushing buttons on the patient's bed and inadvertently raised the height of the bed, while you were attending to another patient. The patient did not use the call bell, attempted to get up to go to the bathroom, and fell. After examination, the patient had a broken femur. The family has initiated a lawsuit for malpractice. Is this case malpractice? Explain your answer.

2. What are the four factors that must be met to be considered malpractice.

3. What is meant by "scope of practice" and what determines the scope? Explain your response.

4. Define the standards of practice.

5. What is the nurse practice act?

6. Explain why a graduate student must pass the state board of nursing exam.

7. Who is the nursing license meant to protect? Explain your rationale.

8. The electrical cord on the bed has exposed wires. Occasionally, a spark can be seen. The patient care technician states, "Your patient complained he received a shock when his foot touched the bed frame and he thinks his life was put in danger. The patient is talking about suing." Who is responsible for the functionality of the equipment used? Explain your response.

9. What is a tort?

10. What is a deposition?

11. What is a defendant?

12. What is a complainant?

13. Explain the process of a medical lawsuit from the initial filing to the result.

14. Define litigation and how does it affect professional nursing.

15. What is a subpoena?

16. What is an affidavit?

LAW WORKSHEET 2

1. Define law.

2. What is the main purpose of a law?

3. What, if any, would be the penalties for violating the law?

4. Define ethics.

5. What is the main purpose of ethics?

6. What, if any would be the penalties for violating ethics?

7. What are moral values?

8. What is the main purpose of moral values?

9. What, if any, would be the penalties for violating moral values?

10. Define protocol.

11. What is the main purpose of protocols?

12. What, if any, would be the penalties for violating protocols?

13. How are the laws enforced by the state board of nursing?

14. Compare the difference between morals and ethics.

15. Define Values.

16. How do morals and values relate to ethics in nursing?

17. How do religious beliefs play a role in ethics?

18. During the Covid-19 pandemic medical supplies were not readily available. A shortage of ventilators was of concern. Who shall be given the use of a ventilator knowing the person not chosen would or could die? Explain your answer.

MAKE-UP ASSIGNMENT 1

1. Explain what evidence-based-practice is and how it pertains to bedside nursing.

2. What is diversity in nursing and how does it play a key role?

3. Must laboratory results be known prior to medication administration? Does pharmacy play a role in this interaction? Explain your response.

4. List three types of nurses that are currently in the nursing profession. Include their unique characteristics in your response.

5. List the various nursing positions or nursing jobs. Include how education plays a role in these various positions.

6. Should nurses get involved in legislation? Include in your response how the state board of nursing plays a role.

7. Explain how euthanasia differs from comfort care.

8. Does the academic arena of nursing differ from bedside nursing in relationship to salaries? Explain your response.

9. It has been stated that, "nursing eats their young." What is the remise to this statement. Do you believe it is true? Explain your response.

10. Should continuing educational units be a mandatory requirement for the nursing profession? Explain your response.

MAKE-UP ASSIGNMENT 2

Research one nursing article (peer-reviewed) that pertains to your chosen field of nursing. Write a summary of the article. Include why this field is your chosen field and how this article supports your choice.

MAKE-UP ASSIGNMENT 3

Make up an examine question for each of the following health disparities.

1. Cerebral vascular accident
2. Closed head injury
3. Myocardial infarction
4. Angina
5. Pneumonia
6. Gastrointestinal bleed
7. Small bowel obstruction
8. Renal failure
9. Pressure ulcers
10. Fractured hip

Match the following work sheet

		Match column 2 with column 1
A. Physiological	a. family	a.
	b. acceptance	b.
	c. sleep	c.

Review Maslow's hierarchy. Match the following

B. Safety and security	d. intimacy	d.
	e. food	e.
	f. achievement	f.
	g. confidence	g.
C. Love and belonging	h. health	h.
	i. breathing	i.
	j. morality	j..
D. Self-esteem	k. shelter	k.
	l. friendship	l.
	m. water	m.
E. Self- actualization	n. job	n.
	o. clothing	o.

MATERNITY 1

Match the following.
1. Creamy appearing breast milk
2. Breast milk that ceases approximately three weeks after the birth of the new born
3. Breast milk that contains 90% water

4. Breast milk that provides immunity for newborn
5. Breast milk that contains lactose and has high levels of fat

Match with definition above and place your answer in the appropriate space below

    A. Colostrum   B. Transitional   C. Mature

1._____ 2._____ 3._____ 4._____ 5._____

- Explain the psychological difference between breast milk and formula in mother- baby bonding.

- Explain what is meant when the milk is letting down.

- Briefly explain how a new mother can determine her baby is obtaining milk when placed to the breast.

MATERNITY 2

1. Briefly compare and contrast cultural breast feeding practices for the following:

    a. Hispanic
    b. Asian
    c. African American

2. List two reasons breast milk production may cease.

3. Can breast milk be refrigerated? If yes, how many days may breast milk be refrigerated and still be considered usable?

4. Can breast milk be frozen? Explain your response.

5. Can the consumption of breast milk cause a change in the color of the baby's stool?

6. Explain the relationship between breast feeding and wet diapers. Include why this relationship is important.

7. A mother must take medication for a sinus infection. Will drugs be present in the breast milk? Explain your response.

8. Can consumed food cause a change in the color of breast milk? Explain your response.

9. Can food and beverages that the mother consumes cause the baby to NOT want to nurse? Explain your response.

MATERNITY 3

1. Briefly describe the stages of labor.

2. Briefly describe the phases of labor.

3. Briefly describe the differences between true labor and false labor.

4. Are there signs that precede labor? Explain your response.

5. Define: latent, active, and transition.

6. What is the difference between internal and external fetal monitoring?

7. Give an example when internal fetal monitoring may be required.

8. Give an example when external fetal monitoring may be required.

9. What is the importance of baseline changes in fetal monitoring?

10. Define: Accelerations as it pertains to fetal monitoring.

11. Briefly explain the difference between early, variable, and late deceleration in fetal monitoring.

12. Explain the difference between voluntary and involuntary uterine contractions.

13. What is uterine fatigue? Include an example of what may cause uterine fatigue.

14. Explain how the mother's position may affect the strength and frequency of contractions.

15. Briefly explain the relationship between hydration and uterine activity

16. List three factors that may influence the pushing efforts of the mother.

MATERNITY 4

1. Define the following:

    a. Fontanels

    b. Breech

c. Transverse

d. Attitude

e. Position

f. Contraction pattern

g. Effacement

h. Cervical dilation

i. Cephalic

2. Name the sutures of the fetus

3. Briefly explain the relationship between the position of fetus and level of pain experienced by the mother.

4. List ways in which the nurse can determine the birth is eminent.

5. List ways in which the nurse may held make the mother more comfortable during labor.

MATERNITY 5

1. Match the following:

To be defined	definition	Correct response

a. Presumptive signs of pregnancy	1. Lack of menses	a._____
b. Probable signs of pregnancy	2. Signs experienced by the woman herself	b._____
c. Positive signs of pregnancy	3. Softening of the cervix	c._____
d. Amenorrhea	4. Signs apparent on physical exam by the doctor	d._____
e. Goodell's sign	5. Bluish vaginal tissue	e._____
f. Chadwick's sign	6. Signs that determine a positive pregnancy	f._____

2. What is supine hypotension syndrome and what intervention must the nurse provide when the woman presents with supine hypotension syndrome?

3. In the table below, list one change that occurs in the pregnant woman

Breast	
Blood volume	
Respiratory	
Gastrointestinal	
Cardiac	
urinary	

MATERNITY 6

Match the word	To the definition	Correct answer
1. Apgar score	a. Vaginal discharge status post (S/P) delivery	1.

	consisting of mucous, blood and tissue	
2. hyperbilirubinemia	b. Flexion of the legs and arms of the infant when startled by loud noise(s)	2.
3. Lochia	c. Incision to avoid tearing or laceration of the perineum	3.
4. Acrocyanosis	d. Elevated levels of insufficient conjugated serum bilirubin	4.
5. Moro's reflex	e. Scale on which the condition of the newborn is assessed immediately after birth	5.
6. Areola	f. Breakdown product of hemoglobin that produces an orange pigment	6.
7. Episiotomy	g. Bluish color of infants hands and feet at the time of birth to 10 days after time of birth	7.
8. Bilirubin	h. Darker tissue surrounding the nipple	8.

MATERNITY 7

POSTPARTUM

1. Briefly explain why the new mother experiences "afterpains" postpartum.

2. Explain the changes in the lochia from rubra, serosa, and alba. Include why quarter size clots should be reported in your response.

3. Why should the breasts be assessed for redness, heat, pain, and engorgement?

4. Why is it important to assess the level of the fundus?

5. What is the purpose of assessing the amount and type of lochia?

6. Your patient who has had an epidural removed complains of a headache. Is a headache normal after the removal of an epidural? Explain your response.

7. You are assessing the fundus and notice it is off-center. What can cause this to occur?

8. Your patient states she heard an old wife's tale that a woman doesn't ovulate when breast feeding and therefore, cannot get pregnant. Is this true? Explain your response.

9. Explain why the doctor maybe concerned that the mother is Rh negative and her baby is Rh positive.

10. Briefly explain which hormone influences milk let down and what action stimulates the hormone.

MATERNITY 8

1. What is meant by maternal-infant attachment?

2. Explain what occurs during the taking-in phase.

3. Explain what occurs during the taking-hold phase.

4. Explain what occurs during the letting-go phase.

5. Your patient returns to for her postpartum check-up. She admits that she noticed significant hair loss. Briefly explain what may cause this to occur.

6. List four ways to resolve hard and tender engorged breast.

7. List ways to help prevent engorgement in the non-breastfeeding mother.

8. Explain the relationship of lactogenesis and the hormones: estrogen, progesterone, prolactin, and oxytocin.

9. List a minimal of four benefits to breastfeeding. (Include both maternal and infant benefits in your response).

10. What is the concern if the patient is diagnosed with uterine atony?

11. List why your patient may experience hypotension.

12. Briefly explain why there is an increased risk of thromboembolism in your postpartum patient.

13. List two reasons breast feeding is contraindicated.

14. What is the purpose of a lactation consultant?

1. List five causes that may inhibit involution status post-delivery.
2. What duration would you expect to see lochia rubra?
3. What duration would you expect to see lochia serosa?
4. What duration would you expect to see lochia alba?
5. There is an offensive odor to the lochia. What may be the cause?
6. What types of analgesia may be used during labor? Include how the analgesia may affect the mother or the infant in your response.
7. Briefly define what is a support person and their role during the labor process.
8. Can the absence of a support person affect the mother who is in labor? Explain your response.
9. How can the fetal heart rate be obtained during labor?
10. How long do contractions continue after the birth of the baby?
11. Define multipara.
12. Define Para.
13. What concerns may present in the laboring substance abuse mother?
14. List two reasons a caesarian birth may be required.
15. What is Lamaze?
16. What is Naegele's rule?
17. Why is it important to complete a cultural assessment?
18. Explain the relationship between late deceleration and fetal distress.

MEDICATION 1

1. List three medication your patient has been prescribed or have your instructor assign three medications. Complete the following for each medication.

Medication name	Classification of each medication listed

Medication name	Indications for each medication

Medication name	Usual dosage of each medication

Medication name	Side effects or adverse reaction of each

2. Your patient has been prescribed a short and long-acting insulin. Complete the following.

Name a short-acting insulin	Name a long-acting insulin

List the onset of the short-acting insulin	List the onset of the long-acting insulin

List the peak time of the short-acting insulin	List the peak time of the long-acting insulin

List one insulin the short-acting insulin can be mixed with and one it cannot be mixed with	List one insulin the long-acting insulin can be mixed with and one it cannot be mixed with

MENTAL HEALTH 1

Word	Match the correct Definition	
1. Repression	A.	a. returning to less developed state
2. Suppression	B.	b. separating from conscious awareness
3. Projection	C.	c. inhibiting feelings
4. Regression	D.	d. justifying
5. Rationalization	E.	e. act of stopping self
6. Disassociation	F	f. attributes given to another
7. Reaction formation	G	g. express opposite of true feelings

Match the following

	1.	a. Believing self is dead
A. grandiose		
B. Delusions	2.	b. Believing self is important
C. Nihilistic	3.	c. believes others are against
D. Persecution	4.	d. False beliefs

77

MENTATL HEALTH 2

Match the following suicidal risk to the correct definition

Level	Correct level	definition
1. high risk	A.	a. The patient has a plan, less likely to elope, past suicidal plans, monitor frequently
2. moderate risk	B.	b. No plan. Zero, one or two symptoms.
3. low risk	C.	c. Patient has a lethal plan. Denies any hope

Fill in the blank from the options from the table below.

1. Desires to be treated as the opposite sex from which the patient has been given at birth. _____.
2. Disturbed thoughts and auditory hallucinations that may be a risk for violence to self or others. _____.
3. May have increased libido, elation, fragmented thoughts, flight of ideas, and change in sleep and appetite. _____.
4. Failure to pay attention. Avoids tasks that are considered disliked. Fails to listen. _____.

A.	Bipolar
B.	Attention deficit disorder
C.	Schizophrenic

D.	Gender dysphoria

MUSCULOSKELETAL 1

1. Define the following and explain its importance in a skeletal injury:
   a. Pain
   b. Pulse
   c. Paresthesia
   d. Paralysis
   e. Pallor
2. List two acute orthopedic emergencies. Explain why they are emergencies.
3. Match the fracture to its definition

Fracture	Definition
1. Open fracture/compound	a. Fracture of bone but bone does not move or misalign
2. Greenstick fracture	b. Fracture that runs horizonal to bone
3. Transverse fracture	c. Fracture resulting with bone breaking through skin.
4. Spiral fracture	d. Fracture of bone but fracture does not extend through bone
5. Non-displaced fracture	e. A twisting motion of bone with fracture

1. _____ 2. _____ 3. _____ 4. _____ 5. _____

5. List three most common reasons for fractures.

a.
b.
c.

4. What are shin splints? Can shin splints develop into fractures? Explain your answer

MUSCULOSKELETAL SYSTEM 2

1. Why is there a concern for compartment syndrome when there is a limb injury?
2. When the patient has been diagnosed with compartment syndrome, what intervention should be implemented?
3. The patient with a compartment syndrome says the doctor instructed him to keep his leg at the level of his heart? The wants to know why. Briefly explain what your answer to this patient would be.
4. What is buck's traction?
5. What type of injury would buck's traction be used for?
6. What is the difference between an open and a closed fracture?
7. What is an immobilizer?
8. What is pin care and how often should it be performed?
9. When should a back brace be applied? With the patient sitting or lying?
10. Briefly explain how a sling should be positioned for the patient with a broken clavicle.
11. What is the risk of immobility when the patient is on strict bedrest.
12. List two benefits of increased mobility for the hospitalized patient.
13. What is deconditioning and how does hospitalization play a role in its potential occurrence as well as its prevention.

14. Briefly explain the relationship between immobility and respiratory complications.

MUSCULOSKELETAL 3

Match the following topic with the correct definition

Topic	definition
1. Scoliosis	a. Genu valgum
2. Kyphosis	b. Dorsal flexion that may be temporary or permanent
3. Foot drop	c. Over curvature of the thoracic vertebra
4. Knock knees	d. Lateral curvature of the spine

1. _____ 2. _____ 3. _____ 4. _____

2. What is an abductor pillow?

3. What condition post operatively would you use an abductor pillow?

4. What could be done if a "baby" toe is broken?

5. What is meant by cast care?

6. Why would it be important for the nurse to assess the pulse and/or skin of the extremity with a cast?

7. Can a patient with a cast take a bath or shower? Explain your response.

8. Should the patient with a broken clavicle, sleep with their sling in place?

9. What is a halo brace?

10. What is a cervical brace and when would it be used?

11. What is whiplash?

12. What is traction and when would it be used.

NEUROLOGY 1

1. List what neurological functions may be assessed in a neurological assessment.

2. List procedures that may be used to determine an ischemic stroke or cerebral aneurysm.
   _____

3. List the purpose of an E.E.G. (electroencephalography). Give two health issues that an E.E.G. may be used to diagnose.
   _____

4. What is intracranial pressure (ICP) monitoring and what are the normal values.
   _____

5. What is the true name of a "spinal tap" and what is its purpose?
   _____
   _____

6. When would a "spinal tap" be contraindicated? Explain your answer.

NEUROLOGY 2

1. What is meningitis?
   _____
   _____.

2. List at minimum two types of meningitis.
   _____
   _____.

3. List two objective signs that when tested are positive in meningitis.

a.	
b.	

4. What procedure can be performed to confirm meningitis?
   _____.

5. List a potential complication of meningitis.
   _____
   _____.

6. What is a seizure?
   _____
   _____.

7. Define epilepsy.
   _____
   _____
   _____.

8. List causes for a seizure.

a.	b.
c.	d.
e.	f.
g.	h.

NEUROLOGY 3

1. Give a brief description of each type of seizure listed below.

SEIZURE	DESCRIPTION
General	
Tonic	
Clonic	
Myoclonic	
Complex	
Simple	

2. List safety precautions for a seizure patient.
   a. _____
   b. _____
   c. _____
   d. _____
   e. _____
   f. _____

3. What patient teaching would you give a seizure patient regarding the following?

ISSUE	TEACHING
Drinking alcohol with antiseizure medication	

Driving and frequent seizure activities	
Antiseizure medication and oral care	
Water and fire safety	

NEUROLOGICAL 4

1. List a symptom of each of the following stages of Parkinson's disease.

STAGE 1	
STAGE 2	
STAGE 3	
STAGE 4	
STAGE 5	

2. List five physical findings that a nurse would observe in a Parkinson's disease patient.
    a. _____
    b. _____
    c. _____
    d. _____
    e. _____

3. Is Alzheimer's disease reversible? Explain your response.

4. List an example of each of the stages of Alzheimer's disease.

Stage 1: normal function	
Stage 2: very mild	
Stage 3: mild	
Stage 4: Moderate	

Stage 5: Moderate severe	
Stage 6: Severe	
Stage 7: Late-Stage	

5. List safety interventions for the Alzheimer's disease patient.
    a. _____
    b. _____
    c. _____
    d. _____
    e. _____

NEUROLOGY 5

1. What is the disease described below?
An autoimmune disease which demonstrates damaged myelinated sheaths in the central nervous system

2. What would bring this patient into the emergency room?

3. Give a nursing diagnosis for this patient.

4. What would be an anticipated medication for this disease?

5. What tests or procedures would you expect for this patient and why?

6. What health care team members would you anticipate would be on this patient's case?

7. What safety interventions should be implemented for this patient?

8. What patient teaching would be needed for this patient. Make certain to cover safety, medication, and mobility in your response.
   _____
   _____
   _____
   _____
   _____.

9. When would you anticipate the patient would be cleared for discharge to home or transferred to a skilled nursing inpatient facility (SNIF)?

   _____

NEUROLOGY 6

1. What is the disease described below?
Disease of upper and lower motor neurons that progress to muscular atrophy, paralysis, then death

2. What would bring this patient into the emergency room?
   _____
   _____.

3. What would be an anticipated medication for this disease?
   _____
   _____.

4. What tests or procedures would you expect for this patient and why?
   _____
   _____.

5. What health care team members would you anticipate would be on this patient's case?
   _____
   _____
   _____
   _____.

6. What safety interventions should be implemented for this patient?
   _____
   _____
   _____.

7. What patient teaching would be needed for this patient. Make certain to cover safety, medication, and mobility in your response.
   _____
   _____

8. When would you anticipate the patient would be cleared for discharge to home or transferred to a skilled nursing inpatient facility (SNIF)?

NEUROLOGY 7

1. What is the disease described below?
Autoimmune disease in which there is a loss of acetylcholine receptors at the neuromuscular junction

2. What would bring this patient into the emergency room?

3. Give a nursing diagnosis for this patient.

4. What would be an anticipated medication for this disease?

5. What tests or procedures would you expect for this patient and why?

6. What health care team members would you anticipate would be on this patient's case?

7. What safety interventions should be implemented for this patient?

8. What patient teaching would be needed for this patient. Make certain to cover safety, medication, and mobility in your response.

9. When would you anticipate the patient would be cleared for discharge to home or transferred to a skilled nursing inpatient facility (SNIF)?

NEUROLOGY 8

1. What characteristics does multiple sclerosis (MS), Amyotrophic lateral sclerosis (ALS), and Myasthenia Gravis (MG) have in common?

2. Explain the difference between relapsing and remission.

3. List a minimum of two risk factors that may trigger a relapse in multiple sclerosis.

4. Which neurosensory disorder may present with Uhthoff's sign?

5. What is Uhthoff's sign?
   _____
   _____.

6. Define the following:
   a. Dysarthria _____
   b. Dysphagia_____
   c. Expressive aphagia _____
   d. Agnosia _____
   e. Neglect _____
   f. Receptive aphagia _____
   g. Hemiplegia _____
   h. Hemiparesis _____

NEUROLOGY 9

1. List two or more reasons a patient may complain of a headache.
   a. _____
   b. _____
   c. _____
   d. _____
   e. _____

2. Define the difference between a migraine and a cluster headache.

Migraine	Cluster headache

3. List the symptoms the patient may complain to have occurred due to a headache.

4. Define the following stages of a headache.

Prodromal	
Aura	
Second stage	
Third stage	
Recovery stage	

5. List actions that may worsen a headache.

Are there foods that might trigger a migraine? If so, explain why and list the food.

NEUROLOGY 10

1. List the different classifications of head injury.

2. List two areas that may bleed from a head injury.

3. When a patient is admitted for a head injury, what other precautions should the nurse take?

4. Explain what is meant by the golden hour when a patient is brought into the emergency room with a head injury.
   _____
   _____
   _____.

5. Why are the cranial nerves tested in a neurological assessment?
   _____
   _____
   _____.

6. When you are assessing your febrile patient, you notice nuchal rigidity. What is nuchal rigidity and what does it indicate?

NEUROLOGY 11

1. What may cause an increase in intracranial pressure?

2. List several interventions that the nurse may implement to reduce intracranial pressure.

3. What is the Monroe-Kellie Doctrine?

4. Explain the process of brain herniation.

NEUROLOGY 12

1. Explain the difference between an embolic stroke versus a hemorrhagic stroke.

2. What does hypercapnia cause in the brain?

3. What happens in the brain when the patient is hyperventilated.

4. Why are stool softeners ordered for patients with a head injury. Explain how intracranial pressure plays a role.

5. Explain the physiological differences between the following and their significance.

Decorticate posturing	
Decerebrate posturing	

6. Explain the difference between the following

Diabetes insipidus	
Syndrome of inappropriate antidiuretic syndrome.	

NEUROLOGY 13

1. Match the following

Hemorrhagic stroke	Clot traveled from the body to cerebral artery
Thrombotic stroke	Arterial rupture
Embolic stroke	Occlusion from an accumulation of platelets and fibrin on an atherosclerotic plaque

2. List two neurological issues that may occur in a patient with a right hemispheric stroke.
   _____
   _____.

3. Define, what is neurogenic shock?

4. Define the following:

Orthostatic hypotension	
Autonomic dysreflexia	
laminectomy	

5. Explain the relationship between sensation and dermatomes.

NEUROLOGY 14

1. Briefly explain the relationship between the cerebrum and the corpus callosum.

2. List the various sections of the left and right lobes.

3. What is the diencephalon?

4. Explain how the cranial nerves may warn of fan impending herniation.

5. Where is cerebral spinal fluid secreted?

6. What is intracranial pressure?

7. Whis is the normal value for intracranial pressure?

8. How does the brain receive its blood supply?

9. What is cerebral perfusion pressure?

10. What is the normal value for cerebral perfusion pressure?

11. Briefly explain what the Monro-Kellie hypothesis is.

12. How does autoregulation occur?

Briefly define the following types of brain injury.

1. Contusion

2. Hematoma

3. Hemorrhage

4. Concussion

5. Diffuse axonal injury

NEUROLOGY 15

Match the following

1. Contusion	A. A blood leak
2. Hematoma	B. Bruises on the parenchyma

3. Epidural hematoma	C. Blood between the skull and the dura mater
4. Subdural hematoma	D. Bleeding between the arachnoid and the pia mater
5. Subarachnoid hemorrhage	E. Collection of blood
6. Intracranial hemorrhage	F. Blood between the dura mater and the arachnoid layer

1. _____ 2. _____ 3. _____ 4. _____ 5. _____ 6. _____

List what may be included in a bedside neurological assessment. (remember to include vital signs)

1. What is a pronator drift?

2. What is the rationale for frequent cranial nerve and pupil assessments in the patient with a head injury.

Define the following and why it is assessed.

1. Corneal reflex

2. Cough reflex

3. Gag reflex

4. Babinski reflex

NEUROLOGY 16

Briefly define the following test/procedure

1. Neurological imaging

2. Intracranial monitoring

3. Cerebral blood flow
4. C.T. scan
5. M.R.I.
6. Angiography

Answer the following:

1. What is the difference between a subarachnoid bolt and an ICP drain?
2. What is a transcranial doppler ultrasonography?
3. What is an electrophysiologic monitoring (EEG)? Give an example when it would be used.
4. What is the end goal in the treatment of the patient with a head injury?
5. What is a transtentorial herniation?
6. Why should the nurse not attempt to place a nasogastric tube in the patient with a basilar skull fracture?
7. Why should hypotonic IV fluids be avoided in the patient with a head injury?
8. When is ICP monitoring considered appropriate?
9. What does it mean if the patient is posturing?
10. Why should hypercapnia be monitored in the patient with a head injury?
11. What occurs when a patient with a traumatic brain injury is hyperventilated?
12. List three medications that maybe used to control intracranial pressure.

NEUROLOGY 17

1. Why should the nurse enforce a low or no stimulation for the traumatic brain injured patient?
2. The patient with a traumatic head injury has been hyperthermic then hypothermic without any intervention. Explain why this occurs.

3. Why must the nurse monitor for the following in the neurologically injured patient?

    a. Vasospasms

    b. Seizures

    c. Intracranial infections

4. Why are anticonvulsants prophylactically prescribed for the traumatic brain injured patient?

5. What are trickle feeds and why are they an important part in the nutritional support in the patient with a traumatic brain injured patient?

Often the nurse must use the following to assess the response of the neurologically injured patient. Briefly describe the following and what it means if there is or isn't a response.

    a. Trapezius pinch

    b. Nail bed pressure

1. List two interventions that a nurse may use to reduce a brain injured patient's ICP.

2. What are battle signs?

3. What are racoon eyes?

4. Which part of the brain has the respiratory control center?

NURSING HISTORY

Match the nurse to the accomplishment

1. Clarissa (Clara) Barton

2. Mary Breckinridge
3. Virginia Henderson
4. Hazel W. Johnson-Brown
5. Mary Eliza Mahoney
6. Florence Nightingale
7. Margaret Sanger
8. Sojourner Truth
9. Dorothea Dix
10. Anna Caroline Maxwell
11. Lillian Ward
12. Jacqueline Fawcett

a. Organized first army nurse corps
b. Founder of American Birth control league which later became planned parenthood
c. Co-founder of the National Association of Colored graduate nurses
d. Activist-advocated for nurse education for African-American nurses
e. Founded first science-based nursing school
f. Founded the Red Cross of America
g. Founded frontier nursing & midwifery

h. Theorist. Shaped nursing education with the nursing need theory
i. Director of Walter Reed. First Afro-American woman general
j. Advocate for better treatment of the mentally ill
k. Pioneered public health nursing in U.S.
l. Expert in nursing conceptual models & theories.

Answer section
1. _____
2. _____
3. _____
4. _____
5. _____
6. _____
7. _____
8. _____
9. _____
10. _____
11. _____
12. _____

NURSING PROCESS 1

1. What is the purpose of the nursing assessment?

2. List three assessment skills needed to perform a thorough assessment.

3. What is subjective data?

4. What is objective data?

5. List 2 sources in which subjective data can be collected.

6. What can be done if there are discrepancies in the subjective data collected?

7. What is intuition and how does it play a role in assessment?

8. What method is used to organize the data collected by the nurse?

9. How does clustering data aid the nurse in determining priority problems?

10. What is an initial assessment?

11. What is a focused assessment?

12. Should an initial assessment be completed each shift? Explain your response.

13. Should a holistic assessment be part of the initial assessment or only focused on the patient? Explain your response.

14. What type of assessment must be completed in an emergent situation?

15. What is a concept map?

16. How does a concept map guide the student?

17. What is a nursing care plan?

18. Is a nursing care plan prepared solely for the use of nurses caring for the patient? Explain your response.

NURSING WORKSHEET 1

1. Explain the difference between dereliction of duty and abandonment. Give an example of each.

2. Should a nursing student or a nurse have malpractice insurance? Explain the pros and cons of having malpractice insurance.

3. A patient or the patient's family may have unrealistic expectations of the care and treatment of the patient. "We saw on the internet this new herbal medication that stops cancer, cures diabetes, and reverses heart failure. Can't you try that?" Explain the response you would give.

4. Define documentation.

5. When must the nurse or other healthcare team members document in the patient's chart?

6. When is it acceptable to document at the end of the shift? (Think emergent situations)

7. You are asked to work in the emergency room. A patient is admitted by ambulance. The patient is in respiratory distress, unconscious, and without family or friend. The doctor orders oxygen, a breathing treatment, and a steroid. Can you administer the steroid without knowing any past medical history or allergy status of the patient? Explain your answer.

8. You are driving home. You see a car accident with the driver pinned behind the wheel. You rush to help. The patient is unconscious. The gas tank has ruptured and the hot motor may ignite the gas at any time. You remove the driver and drag him yards away moments before the car erupts into flame. The patient is later diagnosed with spinal injuries resulting in paralysis due to being removed from the car without a cervical collar or spine support. Explain how the Good Samaritan law will protect you.

9. A patient that was angry with the doctor is discharged. Four years later the patient decides he will sue. Explain what statue of limitations is and does it apply to this scenario. Explain your response.

10. What is administrative law and how does it differ from rules and regulations set forth by the state?

PAIN 1

Match the following

WORD	DEFINITION
1. Modulation	a. Converts painful stimuli to an electrical impulse
2. Transduction	b. The point at which a person feels pain
3. Transmission	c. Move away from a painful stimulus
4. Threshold	d. Traveling of impulses that reduce the intensity of the stimulus
5. Tolerance	e. Level in which the person is willing and able to handle

1._____ 2._____ 3._____ 4._____ 5._____

1. Match the following.

1. Acute pain	a.	Recurrent. Last greater than six months.
2. Chronic pain	b.	Pain from damaged nerves
3. Nociceptive pain	c.	Sudden onset. Temporary. Last less than six months. Usually resolves
4. Neuropathic pain	d.	Pain from damage to or inflammation of tissue(s)

1. _____ 2. _____ 3. _____ 4. _____

2. List causes of the following.

Chronic pain	Acute pain

PAIN 2

104

1. List ways to manage pain. List pharmacological and non-pharmacological methods.

Pharmacological methods	Non-pharmacological methods

2. List what data a nurse may ask a patient regarding the patient's pain.

3. List three types of nociceptive pain.

4. What is COX1 and COX2? How do they differ and how are they similar?

5. How do prostaglandins play a role in pain?

PAIN 3

1. When assessing pain, what does intensity refer to?

2. How would you assess the quality of the patient's pain? What does quality mean?

3. What is a FLACC pain scale?

4. On what type of patient's would the FLACC pain scale be used?

5. List two barriers to effective pain management.

6. Define the following pain scales and on which patient population it would be used.

SCALE	DEFINE/POPULATION
NIPS	
WONG-BAKER	
CRIES	
FLACC	
NUMBER	
BEHAVIORAL	

7. Why is so difficult to manage pain in a patient with a substance abuse problem?

8. What is meant by a comprehensive pain assessment?

9. What is a common physical complication of narcotic usage?

10. Can pain be controlled completely? Explain your response.

PAIN 4

1. What is epidural pain management and what does it target?

2. What are the benefits of epidural pain management?

3. What concerns or side effects may occur with epidural pain management?

4. What is the difference between acute pain and chronic pain?

5. How can pain be assessed and managed in the non-verbal patient?

6. Is there a difference between opioid dependence and addiction? Explain your response.

7. What is complex regional pain syndrome?

8. Explain how untreated pain may affect the immune system.

Match the following.

1. Acute pain	a. Pain that last beyond expected healing duration
2. Chronic pain	b. Precepted pain caused by increased response to stimuli
3. neuropathic pain	c. short duration with identifiable cause
4. allodynia	D. increased pain caused by stimulation that is normally not a painful sensation
5. hyperalgesia	e. pain due to damage to nerve(s)

9. Explain why subjective pain assessments may be difficult?

10. List the seven elements that should be included in a pain assessment.

PAIN 5

1. Why shouldn't the patient be given unrealistic pain control expectations?

2. List five behaviors that may indicate pain.

1.	
2.	
3.	
4.	
5.	

3. Explain how a pain scale can be objectively used to assess pain.

4. Can pain be assessed in the intubated pain? Explain your response.

5. Why is it difficult to assess pain in the patient with a history of drug abuse?

6. What is an opioid risk tool and why or when should it be used?

7. What is an analgesic ladder?

8. What is considered mild pain?

9. What is considered moderate pain?

10. What is considered severe pain?

11. List four factors that play a role in determining drug addiction.

PAIN 6

1. Explain how opioids bind to mu, kappa, and delta sites.

2. Can genetic variability affect opioid effectiveness? Explain your response.

3. What is intrathecal pain control?

4. What is a nerve block?

5. What is a Q-pump?

6. What is a PCA?

7. Why is there a concern for the PCA by proxy?

8. Briefly explain what a multimodal analgesic regime is and why it can enhance pain relief.

9. What is a narcotic?

10. How should narcotics be disposed?

11. When a narcotic is ordered, why should the lowest dose be given instead of the highest dose?

12. List two medications that may potentiate the effectiveness of a narcotic.

13. List two medications that may considered antagonist of a narcotic.

14. What does it mean to potentiate?

15. What does it mean to be an antagonist medication?

16. List three other interventions that may assist with pain relief in conjunction with the administration of the pain medication.

17. List two narcotics that may be given in oral, intramuscular, and IV form.

18. How long does it take an intramuscular pain medication to begin working?

PAIN SCALES

Match the following pain scale with their description

Pain tool	Description	Correct match
A. Numeric scale	1. Used in critical care areas to assess pain based on observation	a.
B. N-Pass scale	2. Assessment for advanced dementia patients	b.
C. FLACC scale	3. (9 year old to elderly) Assessed via perceived level of pain	c.
D. FACES scale	4. Observational tool used for critical care	d.
E. CRIES scale	5. (Infant to 7 years) observation based tool	e.
F. Behavioral scale	6. Wong-Baker scale for 3 years (plus)	f.
G. CPOT scale	7. Scale for babies 8 months to 16 months	g.
H. PAINAD	8. Scale used for neonates	h.

Mark the behaviors that maybe observed in the cognitively impaired patient experiencing pain.

- o Moaning
- o Guarding
- o Thrashing
- o Sleeping calmly
- o Shallow respirations
- o Frequent moving

PATIENT CARE WORKSHEET 1

1. The nurse must promote a supportive and safe environment. Patients often fear their pain will not be addressed effectively. List ways the nurse can ensure the patient's pain is assessed and pain control measures are implemented. (Include patient education.)

2. Explain how trust plays a key role in patient education

3. Pain is considered the sixth vital sign. List the various types of pain scales available. Give an example of what type or age of the patient the nurse would use for each pain scale.

4. When assessing pain, what data would the nurse need to know prior to calling the doctor for a pain medication?

5. Explain why it is important to know the patient's previous medical history.

6. Why is it important to complete a head-to-toe assessment on a patient within 24 hours of admission?

7. What is the importance of assessing the patient's skin daily?

8. Explain the necessity of reading the previous nurses notes.

9. When should patient education begin? Explain your answer.

10. What is the best way to assess the patient's genitals without embarring the patient?

11. Can the patient refuse to be assessed? Explain your answer.

12. Why is it important to orient the patient to the room?

13. Your patient decides he doesn't want to stay in the hospital. You know he needs more medical care. Does your patient have the right to leave? Explain your answer.

14. What does AMA stand for?

PATIENT CARE WORKSHEET 2

1. You are working in the emergency room. A child is brought in with an elevated temperature. You notice a lot of bruises on the child. Do you need to explain to the parents that you need to make out a report for child abuse? Explain your answer.

2. List the signs that may present in a patient that has been abused.

3. List the signs that may be present in a patient that is neglected.

4. Your shift in the emergency room has not ended. An adolescent comes in and requests treatment for venereal disease. Can you treat this patient or do you require parental consent? Explain your answer.

5. You are assigned a suicidal adolescent who is having difficulty in breathing. He doesn't want any medical intervention. He says, "I just want to die. Leave me alone." What interventions, if any, would you do?

6. The doctor wants your suicidal adolescent admitted to the mental health ward. The patient is refusing. Describe how you would explain the difference between voluntary and involuntary commitment to your patient.

7. What is the difference between a chronic disease and an acute disease. Include an example of each.

8. You have been assigned as a preceptor for a new nurse. Explain how you will teach critical judgement.

9. What is good faith reporting?

10. Your orientee has made a medication error. What should you do? Explain your response.

11. Nosocomial infections are always waiting to happen. What can you, as a health care professional do to help prevent the spread of a nosocomial infection?

12. Your orientee asks you, "What is evidence-based-practice?" How will you respond?

PATIENT CARE WORKSHEET 3

Determine which response is true or false regarding patient rights and responsibility

YES	NO	RESPONSE
		1. Receive respect and efficient care
		2. No need to know their diagnosis
		3. Receive informed consent after the treatment
		4. Not allowed to refuse treatment
		5. Maintain confidentiality
		6. Examine their bill for charges incurred
		7. Can decide if wants to follow physician's instruction
		8. Provide past medical history
		9. Determine if services should be paid
		10. Provided privacy

Using the responses provided above, list which is a patient right and which is a patient responsibility.

1. _____
2. _____
3. _____
4. _____
5. _____
6. _____
7. _____
8. _____
9. _____
10. _____

1. Does the unwritten agreement between a patient and the doctor end completely after the patient had been rendered care and the bill paid? Explain your response.

2. Can the physician cease care if the patient is non-compliant with the ordered regime? Explain your response.

PEDIATRICS 1

1. Explain the relationship between premature infants and lack of the physical development of the various body systems.

2. List a physical issue that may present in a premature male infant.

3. Explain the reflex problems that occur when attempting to feed a premature infant.

4. Briefly explain why premature infants have respiratory issues. Include in your response how surfactant plays a role in this issue.

5. Explain why heat loss is a major concern in the premature infant. Include in your response, two interventions that the nurse may use to help prevent heat loss.

6. What type of issues may present in the infant of diabetic mother.

7. List two factors that may occur to the placenta during pregnancy and how it would influence the growth or survival of the fetus.

8. Define brown fat and its purpose.

9. Define respiratory distress syndrome and its etiology.

Match the following.

	Definition	Correct response
1. Moro reflex	When infant cheek touched, the infant searches for a nipple in attempt to feed	
2. Palmer reflex	When lateral foot stroked, the big toe moves upward and the toes fan outward	
3. Rooting reflex	Infant grasps finger when placed in the hand	
4. Babinski reflex	Infant placed supine & downward extends then abducts extremities	

PEDIATRICS 2

Match the age with the developmental milestone

1. Two months old	Rolls over
2. Four months old	runs
3. Six months old	Holds cup
4. Nine months old	undresses self
5. Twelve months old	crawls
6. Eighteen months old	sits
7. Two years old	smiles
8. Three years old	Rolls over

1. _____ 2. _____ 3. _____ 4. _____ 5. _____ 6. _____ 7. _____ 8. _____

A. List two types of infant injuries that are commonly seen. Include how they could be prevented in your response.

B. What is separation anxiety?

C. List two types of toddler injuries that are commonly seen. Include how they could be prevented in your response.

D. What is parallel play?

PEDIATRICS 3

Complete the following with the timeline of when the vaccines should be administered.

Hepatitis A	
Hepatitis B	
Rotavirus	
DTAP	
Polio	
Varicella	
MMR	
Influenza	

Define the following.

1. Celiac's disease

2. Short bowel syndrome

3. Cleft palate

4. Cleft lip

5. Spina bifida

A. What physical findings would you expect to observe in an infant with increased intracranial pressure?

B. What is shaken baby syndrome? Include in your response signs you would observe if this occurred.

C. What is a febrile seizure?

RESPIRATORY 1

1. Define the following. Explain when it may be ordered.

PFT	
ABG	
Bronchoscopy	
Thoracentesis	
Pulse oximetry	
Nebulizer treatment	

2. Why must an Allen's test be completed before an ABG is performed?
   _____
   _____.

3. In what position should the nurse place the patient when a thoracentesis will be performed?

4. List reasons that may result in in inaccurate pulse oximetry readings.

5. What is the purpose of a chest tube?

6. When should a chest tube be removed?

RESPIRATORY 2

1. A chest tube drainage system has three chambers. Name and list the purpose of each chamber.

_____ _____ chamber	
_____ _____ chamber	
_____ _____ chamber	

2. Explain how the nurse can confirm there is an air leak in the chest tube system.

3. How can the nurse assess the cause of an air leak?

4. What is a sucking chest wound and what might be its cause?

5. What action should the nurse take if a chest tube is accidently disconnected?

6. What does it mean if the fluid in the water seal chamber rises and falls when the patient is breathing normally? Should the doctor be notified?

RESPIRATORY 3

1. Listed are six non-invasive oxygen delivery devices. List how much oxygen each deliver.

Nasal cannula	
Simple mask	
Venturi mask	
Face tent	
Non-rebreather	
BIPAP	

2. What is oxygen toxicity and how does it occur?

3. What is an endotracheal tube?

4. Define the difference between the following.

BIPAP	CPAP	Mechanical ventilation

5. Your patient's ventilator alarm keeps alarming because your patient has a leak in the endotracheal tubes balloon. Can you turn off the ventilator alarm to allow your patient to get some sleep? Explain your answer.

RESPIRATORY 4

1. Define the following.

Word	Define
Cyanosis	
Hypoxemia	
Hypoventilation	
PEEP	
Acidosis	
Alkalosis	
VAP	
Barotrauma	
Atelectasis	
Pleural effusions	
ARDS	
Wheezes	
Crackles	
Rales	

Rhonchi	

2. What is a stridor?

_____

_____

RESPIRATORY 5

1. Match the following ventilator settings to their definition

Ventilator setting	definition
Assist control ventilation	Preset rate and tidal volume that will be given. Patient may breathe spontaneously in between set rate.
Synchronized intermittent mandatory ventilation	The ventilator adds pressure at the end of each breath to keep the alveoli open to promote gas exchange
Pressure support ventilation	Preset rate and tidal volume. Patient may initiate the breath but ventilator delivers the tidal volume for each breath taken. Client may breathe above set rate
Positive end expiratory pressure	Patient initiates rate and tidal volume but assistance is given by the ventilator during inspirations

2. Explain the difference between rhinitis and a common cold.

Rhinitis.	Common cold

3. What is the relationship between pneumonia and influenzas? _____

4. What is the difference between an epidemic and a pandemic?

Epidemic	pandemic

RESPIRATORY 6

1. In a patient diagnosed with pneumonia, what findings would you expect to see in the following?

WBC	
ABG	
SPUTUM SPECIMEN	
BLOOD CULTURES	

2. A Patient with a history of asthma begins to wheeze. Should you be concerned? Explain your response.

_____
_____
_____.

3. List the four categories of asthma.

Category 1	
Category 2	
Category 3	
Category 4	

4. List four triggers of asthma.

5. What is status asthmaticus?

6. You notice your patient has been having labored breathing is showing signs of sternal retraction. What does sternal retractions indicate?

RESPIRATORY 7

1. Define the following. List a known cause of each.

Disease	Definition	cause
COPD		
Emphysema		
Bronchitis		

2. Which respiratory disease may present with a barrel chest?
   _____.

3. What is incentive spirometry and what is its use in a patient with a respiratory disease?
   _____
   _____.

4. List a non-respiratory response of a bronchodilator medication.
   _____.

5. When the nurse instructs the patient to "smell the flowers (slowly inhale) and blow out the candles (slowly exhale)," this practice is to teach to the patient to do what?
   _____
   _____.

6. What is T.B.?
   _____.

7. What pathogen can be seen in a patient diagnosed with T.B.?
   _____.

8. What type of isolation should a patient with active T.B. be placed?
   _____
   _____.

Does T.B. only affect the lungs? Explain your response.

_____

RESPIRATORY 8

1. What is another name for an intradermal test?
   _____
   _____.

2. Define the following different ways to test for T.B.

Mantoux tests	
Quantiferon test	
AFB test	

3. What type of mask should a nurse wear when caring for a patient with active TB?
   _____.

4. When a Mantoux test is administered, when should the results be read?
   _____.

5. Determine the results of the following Mantoux readings.

Results	Population	Positive or negative

124

"0" mm	Nursing assistant	
Less than "5" mm	A patient with no risk factors	
Greater than "5"mm	A HIV positive patient	
Greater than "10" mm	A patient with no risk factors	
Greater than "10"mm	A patient who uses DOA	
Greater than "15"mm	A patient with no risk factors	
Greater than "15"mm	A patient with allergies	

6. A patient has a history of T.B. The patient has been taking the prescribed medication for 11 months. Does this patient require isolation? Explain your response.

___

___

___

___

RESPIRATORY 9

1. Define the following, when they might occur, and the cause.

Pulmonary emboli	
Pleurisy	
Pleural friction rub	

2. What is an IVC filter?

___

___.

3. Define the following and how they relate to a PE.

Test/procedure/symptom	Define	How relates to a PE
Embolectomy		
VQ scan		

PET scan		
Petechiae		

4. What interventions can be done for the patient with a PE? (Remember medications)
_____
_____
_____

RESPIRATORY 10

1. What is the difference between a pneumothorax (PTX) and a hemothorax?
_____
_____
_____
_____
_____.

2. Define the following and how it relates to a PTX.

	Define	How it relates to a PE
Bleb		
Flail chest		
Tracheal deviation		

3. List symptoms of respiratory distress.

4. When a tracheal deviation occurs, in which direction does it deviate?
   _____
   _____.

5. Define the difference between an external and internal PTX.
   _____
   _____.

6. What is a sucking chest wound?

RESPIRATORY 11

1. Explain the pathophysiology of how asthma occurs.

2. Explain why the doctor would order a nebulizer treatment for an asthmatic patient. What does a nebulizer treatment do?

3. List three initial interventions that may be used on an asthmatic patient. Explain your rationale for each intervention.

127

4. Your asthmatic patient states he has been using his inhalers as ordered. How can you be certain the patient is using his inhalers correctly? Explain your response.

5. Explain how you would teach your patient how to use an inhaler. How can you be certain your patient understands the instructions correctly? Explain your response.

RESPIRATORY 12

1. Where would you auscultate and find the following?

Sounds	Location
Bronchial lung sounds	
Bronchovesicular lung sounds	
Vesicular lung sounds	

2. What is adventitious breath sounds and what would be their cause(s)?

3. List 4 different pulmonary diseases and what lung sounds you would hear with each.

4. Describe techniques for auscultating lung sounds.

5. Identify why it is important to auscultate the lungs prior and after performing nasotracheal suctioning.

6. If your patient had a lobectomy, would it be necessary to auscultate for lung sounds over the "missing" lung site? Explain your response.

7. Your patient's son insists his mother (your patient) do abdominal breathing only while awake. What is abdominal breathing?

8. How would you respond to the patient's son?

9. Your patient has Raynaud's disease and the pulse oximetry placed on her finger shows a pulse oximetry level of 58%. What would be your next actions to ensure adequate oxygenation.

SPINAL 1

1. Explain why the loss of functional ability is determined by the level of injury to the spinal cord.
2. Why is immobilization important when a spinal injury occurs?
3. Define autonomic dysreflexia?
4. What is spinal shock?
5. At what level of injury would the patient's ability to breath independently be compromised?
6. List the potential health concerns a male patient may have if diagnosed with paralysis below the waist.
7. What does it mean if the patient is quadriplegic?
8. What does it mean if the patient is paraplegic?
9. If the doctor tells the patient his severity of injury is complete, what does it mean?

10. If the doctor tells the patient his severity of injury is incomplete, what does it mean?

11. Explain why a patient with a spinal cord injury may no longer have control over his bowels or bladder.

12. How can a spinal cord injury affect sexual function?

13. Explain why a paraplegic may have muscle atrophy of the lower extremities.

14. What fears may a quadriplegic patient express? (Hint: think power failure and fire)

15. Is it possible for a paraplegic woman to become impregnated and give birth? Explain your response.

16. List the various types of equipment a patient with a permanent spinal cord injury may require. Note the purpose of each listed equipment.

STATE BOARD REVIEW PRACTICE 1

Using the tables below, choose the most appropriate response.

Your Parkinson's patient's wife asks you how is Parkinson diagnosed. You explain _____.

Table A
1. With a computed tomography (CT) scan
2. By presenting symptoms, family observations, and past medical history
3. Magnetic resonance imaging (MRI) scan

The patient's wife then asks, "How long will it take to cure my husband of this Parkinsons?" You reply _____.

Table B

1. With exercise, diet and medication, it may resolve within four months
2. Every patient responds differently to treatment. It cannot be predicted
3. Symptoms can be managed with medication. Parkinsons disease is a progressive disease with no cure

The patient's wife asks, "Is there anything I should be made aware of when caring for my husband?"

You reply _____.

Table C
1. He may have swallowing issues as the disease progresses. He may choke.
2. People may point and stare when his tremors worsen.
3. There are no concerns to worry about.

STATE BOARD REVIEW PRACTICE 2

Using the tables below, choose the most appropriate response.

Your patient asks you what is Alzheimer's disease. You explain _____.

Table A
4. A progressive neurodegenerative disease
5. A disease that only affects the elderly who are older than 70 years and sickly
6. A communicable disease that can be spread by respiratory droplets

The patient then asks, "What are the risk factors?" You reply _____.

Table B

131

4. Daily exercise, low fat diet, and low carbohydrate intake
5. Low cholesterol, hypoglycemia, and low blood pressure
6. Hypertension, diabetes, obesity, smoking, and hyperlipidemia

The patient asks, "Are there any signs?"

You reply _____.

Table C
4. Forgetfulness, memory loss, and difficulty with words
5. Able to flawlessly recall long-term memory and short-term memory information
6. Begins to take a higher interest in completing routine tasks

STATE BOARD REVIEW PRACTICE 3

Using the tables below, choose the most appropriate response.

Your patient asks you what is Lou Gerig's disease. You explain _____.

Table A
7. A disease known as "dropsy". Labeled after a cherry picker.
8. A disease that causes loss of motor neurons. Labeled after a baseball player.
9. A disease resulting in repetitive speech. Labeled after a radio host.

The patient then asks, "Are there early signs?" You reply _____.

Table B

7. Slurred speech, weakness, and tripping.
8. "Second sight" and hyper-reflexive grasps.
9. Manic episodes with surges of nervous energy.

The patient asks, "Is there a cure?"

You reply _____.

Table C
1. With an implanted deep-brain stimulator.
7. Medications that increase the production of Glutamate.
8. Non-curable degenerative neuromuscular disease

STATE BOARD REVIEW PRACTICE 4

Using the tables below, choose the most appropriate response.

Your patient asks you can he recover from a brain tumor. You explain _____.

Table A
10. The prognosis would depend on the type of tissue, location, and intervention.
11. Absolutely. Medicine has achieved a lot of success with laser surgeries.
12. Yes. Brain tumors are slow growing and can be reduced with radiation therapy.

The patient then asks, "What are the signs of a brain tumor?" You reply _____.

Table B

10. Rigid stance with an inability to bend at the waist.
11. Headaches that worsen at night.
12. Inability to tolerate spicy odors

The patient asks, "how do you test for a brain tumor?"

You reply _____.

Table C
2. An extensive neurological examination and past medical history.
3. By obtaining a mammogram with contrast
4. By using a tuning fork. Striking the tuning fork and touching the center lower jaw

TEST YOUR KNOWLEDGE 1

Define the following:

1. Sediment
2. Donning
3. Ashen
4. Dusky
5. Pallor
6. Ruberous
7. Cyanotic
8. Edema
9. Dehiscence
10. Hyperthermia

Define the following abbreviations:

1. PVD
2. CHF
3. MI
4. CVA
5. MVC
6. JVD
7. SC
8. IM

TEST YOUR KNOWLEDGE 2

1. Explain the difference between an AV graft and an AV fistula.
2. If a patient's A1C is greater than 7, would this confirm the patient was compliant with her diabetic regime? Explain your response.
3. Explain how each of the following topics are complications of diabetes.
    a. Macular degeneration
    b. Neuropathy
    c. Hair loss
4. List the interventions for each of the following basic care and comfort issues.
    a. Hygiene

    b. Progressive mobility

    c. Nutrition

    d. Pain control

5. Why is it important to have an advanced directive?

6. What is a bruit and thrill?

7. What sign is positive when tested for the patient with a diagnosis of meningitis?

8. What is myelopathy?

9. Why is it important to know the chain of command?

10. What equipment should every nurse have readily available daily?

TEST YOUR KNOWLEDGE 3

1. Define encephalitis and potential causes.

2. List three clinical symptoms that may present in the patient with encephalitis. Include one laboratory result in your response.

3. What is Reyes syndrome and what population of patients is it most commonly seen?

4. Define Sepsis.

5. Are there early signs of sepsis that can be monitored for to assist to prevent it from becoming severe? Explain your response.

6. What does it mean to pan culture the patient?

7. What is a seizure? Include two causes of seizures.

8. What is status epilepticus?

9. What is autism? Include how it is diagnosed in your response.

10. What is the difference between cardiomegaly and cardiomyopathy?

11. What is meningitis?

12. What is Kerning's sign?

13. Explain the relationship between epilepsy and seizures.

14. What is Cerebral palsy? Include potential causes in your response.

15. Define the following:

    a. Ataxia
    b. Nystagmus
    c. Decerebrate
    d. decorticate

URINARY SYSTEM 1

Match the following

Fill in the blank

1. Dark urine indicates _____.
2. Pale urine indicates _____.

Polyuria	The retention of waste and metabolites
Oliguria	Leukocytes in the urine
Proteinuria	Elimination of large amounts of urine
Glucosuria	Sign of incomplete fat metabolism
Ketonuria	Exceeds blood glucose reabsorption capability
Hematuria	Urine output of 400 ml or less daily
Pyuria	Protein in the urine
Azotemia	Red blood cells in the urine

3. Rust colored urine indicates _____.
4. The urine will have a fruity odor if _____ are present.
5. Specific gravity is normally _____ to _____.

List the three phases of acute renal failure.

a.

b.

c.

List three pre-renal failure causes.

a.

b.

c.

URINARY SYSTEM 2

1. List three causes of chronic renal failure.

138

a.
   b.
   c.

2. Explain why acidosis occurs when the kidneys fail.

3. Explain why anemia is prevalent in chronic renal failure.

4. Explain what is erythropoietin and its role in renal failure?

5. Define osteomalacia and explain its relationship to renal failure.

6. What is uremic frost?

7. List a nursing intervention for a patient in renal failure with uremic frost.

8. Why must a patient in renal failure have to be concerned about their cardiac status. Explain your response.

9. Your patient has been diagnosed with renal failure. The patient asks, "what is dialysis? The doctor said I will need to have it." Explain what is dialysis and how would you explain it to your patient.

10. Explain why monitoring intake and output is important when caring for a patient in renal failure.

URINARY SYSTEM 3

Define the following:

1. Nephrostomy
2. Nephrectomy
3. Nephrolithotomy
4. Pyelolithotomy
5. Ureterolithotomy
6. Extracorporeal lithotripsy
7. Cystitis
8. Urethritis
9. Extropy of the bladder
10. Ileal conduit
11. Ureterostomy
12. Dialysis

Answer the following questions

1. Why is intake and output important in the renal failure patient?
2. Why must the patient be taught about dietary changes?
3. Why are laboratory results needed more often in the renal patient?
4. Why is it anticipated that the renal patient will become anemic?

URINARY 4

1. List four processes or systems that allow the body to maintain a water balance.

2. Osmoreceptors in which organ is responsible to stimulate thirst and antidiuretic hormone (ADH) from the posterior pituitary?

3. Which section of the kidneys does ADH act upon?

4. Briefly explain what may be the body's main protection against dehydration and hyperosmolarity?

5. List three factors that may influence the secretion of ADH or the thirst mechanism.

6. Explain why the sedated post-surgical patient is at greater risk for a fluid deficit.

7. Explain why a dry mouth does not necessarily indicate a fluid deficit.

8. List two functions of the kidneys.

9. List two health issues that may occur if the kidneys are not functioning properly.

Determine which response below pertains to cortisol or aldosterone

RESPONSE	CORTISOL OR ALDOSTERONE
1. Responds to psychological stressors	
2. Responds to hypotension	
3. Anti-inflammatory effect	
4. Enhances sodium retention	
5. Secreted during the circadian rhythm	

URINARY 5

1. Why do burns cause trouble for the kidneys?

2. Does the geriatric patient have structural changes in the kidneys? Explain your response.

3. Why are women more prone to urinary tract infections? Include one way to decrease or prevent these urinary tract infections.

4. Define hypospadias and include potential health issues that may occur with this condition.

5. Define epispadias and include potential health issues that may occur with this condition.

List why the following urine specimens would be ordered.

DEFINE	RESPONSE
1. Routine urine specimen	
2. Sterile urine specimen	
3. Clean catch or mid-stream urine specimen	
4. Glucose, acetone, and protein in the urine specimen	
5. 24-hour urine specimen	

VITAL SIGNS 1

1. What is the difference between signs and symptoms? Give an example of each.

2. What is Korotkoff?

3. Define the following which can be considered vital signs and their importance.

a. Blood pressure	
b. Heart rate	
c. Respiratory rate	
d. Temperature	
e. Pulse oximetry	
f. Pain	

4. List the various ways the items listed below can be measured.

a. Blood pressure	
b. Heart rate	
c. Respiratory rate	
d. Temperature	
e. Pain	

5. What is pulse pressure and why is it important to know?

6. What is an apical pulse?

VULNERABLE POPULATION PROJECT

Research the following and put together a power point, spread sheet, or research paper.

1. Who are the vulnerable populations in your community? What obstacles do they face? What resources are available? How can they access those resources? What health and safety risks do they face?

2. How do the immigrants assimilate into the community? What obstacles do they face? What resources are available? How do they access those resources? What health and safety risks do they face?

3. Are there homeless people in your community? Where to they eat and sleep? What obstacles do they face? What resources are available? How do they access those resources? Include safety issues for the homeless as well as the local residents. What health and safety risks do they face?

4. What are the age and gender of those at the poverty level in your community? What health risks do they face? What additional issues may they have? (example: buy prescriptions or food). What may be the underlying cause of their poverty? (death of spouse, health decline, etc.).

5. How does your community assist those individuals with mental illness with no means of support (family, friends, or financial)? What health and safety risks do they face?

Choose (a minimum of) one group from above. Critically think how you could help resolve their obstacles. Include what resources you would use. How would you implement this plan of care?

WORD DEFINITIONS 1

Define the following:

#	Term	Definition
1.	TYMPANIC	
2.	ORTHOPNEA	
3.	STETHOSCOPE	
4.	AXILLA	
5.	CYANOSIS	
6.	HYPERETENSION	
7.	NURSING PROCESS	
8.	FOLEY	
9.	ISOLATION	
10.	CHRONIC	
11.	ACUTE	
12.	PALPATION	
13.	SPHYGMOMANAOMETER	
14.	EUPNEA	
15.	TUBE FEEDING	
16.	COGNITIVE	
17.	SEDIMENT	
18.	INTERVENTIONS	
19.	DYSPNEA	
20.	OCCULT BLOOD	
21.	PAIN SCALE	
22.	TRANSFUSION	
23.	LANGUAGE BARRIER	
24.	HYPOTENSION	
25.	APEX	
26.	EDEMA	
27.	DON	
28.	DOFF	
29.	APNEA	
30.	HYPERTHERMIA	

WORK SHEET – LABORATORY

Match the following

1.	WBC – ELEVATED
2.	HgB - ELEVATED
3.	PLT - LOW
4.	POTASSIUM - ELEVATED
5.	SODIUM - ELEVATED
6.	WBC – LOW
7.	BUN – ELEVATED
8.	HgB – LOW

A.	Neurological confusion
B.	Anemia
C.	Infection
D.	Potential for hemorrhage
E.	Potential for cardiac arrest
F.	Dehydration
G.	Cancer
H.	Renal failure

1. _____. 2. _____. 3. _____. 4. _____. 5. _____. 6. _____.
7. _____. 8. _____.

Match the following

1.	Sodium
2.	Potassium
3.	Calcium
4.	Bicarb
5.	Magnesium

a. low level in a drug overdose
b. low levels seen in torsades
c. reduced by diuretics
d. Chvostek's sign seen with low levels
e. Low levels seen with SIADH

1. _____. 2. _____. 3. _____. 4. _____. 5. _____.

WORKSHEET – BEST PRACTICES

1. What is the best position to place the patient for the nurse to assess for jugular vein distention (JVD)?

a. 90 degrees	b. Trendelenburg
c. 45 degrees	d. prone

   Answer: _____

2. If having difficulty auscultating the heart. What position can the patient be placed to assist to better hear the heart sounds?

a. Sitting up, leaning on over the bed table	b. Lying flat, positioned on right side
c. Lying flat, positioned on left side	d. Lying flat, in supine position

   Answer: _____

3. The patient is a quadriplegic. What areas would be prone to pressure ulcers? Mark all that apply

a. Scapula	b. vertebra	c. Anterior wrists
d. Elbows	e. Lateral shoulders	f. Medial ankles
g. Hips	h. Sacrum	i. Medial knees
j. Lateral knees	k. Heels	l. knuckles

   Answer(s): _____.

4. The patient is lying flat in a supine position. The patient complains (C/O) difficulty in breathing. What is the FIRST action you could and should do?

   Answer: _____.

5. What is the first action the nurse should do before entering a patient's room?

   Answer: _____.

WORKSHEET – INTAKE AND OUTPUT

The following are items of measure that the patient had during your shift. Calculate the intake and output and tally for your 8 hour shift.

Jello	6 ounces
Coffee	8 ounces
Bouillion	8 ounces
Urine output	240 ml
IV fluids	50 ml/Hr
IV piggyback	100 ml
Jello x 2	12 ounces
Tea	8 ounces
Water	500 ml
Urine output	650 ml
Emesis	100 ml

Total intake: _____ Total output: _____

Based on your calculations, is the patient euvolemic, hypervolemic, or hypovolemic?

Answer: _____

What is the total difference between the total intake and the total output?

Answer: _____.

List what may be the cause of your difference in intake and output.

URINARY SYSTEM 3

Define the following urinary issues. Specify if it is an infection or a renal condition. compare the difference between acute and chronic, or listed issue, when applicable.

Condition or infection	Define	Compare	How is this issue diagnosed
1. Acute pyelonephritis		Chronic pyelonephritis	
2. Acute glomerulonephritis		Chronic glomerulonephritis	
3. Polycystic kidney		Renal calculi	
4. Renal artery stenosis		Ureteral stricture	
5. Renal calculi			
6. Ureteral stricture			
7. Renal tuberculosis			

WORKSHEET – CLINICAL

1. Record your patient's vital signs in the box

2. Is the patient's systolic blood pressure within normal limits (WNL)?

3. Calculate your patient's mean arterial pressure (MAP). _____

4. Is the MAP adequate or is it too high or too low? _____

5. What are the concerns if the MAP is too high or too low? _____

6. Calculate your patient's pulse pressure. _____

7. Is your patient's pulse pressure WNL, narrow, or wide? _____

8. What are the normal parameters of pulse pressure? _____

9. What are the normal parameters of a heart rate? _____

10. Is your patient's heart rate too high or too low? _____

11. What are the normal parameters of the respiratory rate? _____

12. What is the concern of tachypnea or bradypnea? (hint- pH level) _____.

13. What is the concern of an elevated temperature? _____

14. List reasons the pulse oximetry may not read accurately?
_____
_____.

The following pages are next-gen and critical thinking scenarios

CHEST PAIN next-gen scenario

A 42 year-old male is admitted with chest pain (CP) secondary to coronary artery disease (CAD). Past medical history (PMH): hypertension (HTN), obesity, and smokes 2 packs per day (PPD). The patient is not married and is a long-haul truck driver. Weight: 260 lb. height: 5' 8".

Place the following in the appropriate column.

	Modifiable factors	Non-modifiable factors
Age		
Gender		
Diet		
Weight		
Smoking		
Mobility		
Race		

The patient smokes 2 PPD. How many packs per year does this patient smoke? Choose the correct number from the list below.

	total of Packs per year
52	
730	
104	
365	

NURSE NOTE

Patient drove self to the emergency room (ER). He had accompanied his friend to the gym. After 30 minutes of strenuous exercise, the patient began to experience chest pain. Pain was a 6/10 on the number scale. Patient admits to smoking 2 PPD, drinks 4 – 6 beers daily. Because he is on the road so much, he doesn't cook. He orders fast food for each meal. Lungs CTA. Heart regular, obese. Positive bowel sounds. Voids without difficulty. 1+ edema in bilateral lower extremities.

DOCTOR ORDERS

1. Admit to coronary care unit
2. Nitroglycerin SL now and Q5min. X 3
3. Oxygen at 2 L/min. via NC. Keep pulse oximetry 88 -92 %
4. Continuous cardiac monitor
5. Continuous pulse oximetry
6. EKG
7. 2-D echo
8. NPO
9. Cardiology consult
10. Bedrest
11. VS Q1H
12. Aspirin 325 mg, chew stat
13. Nitroglycerin IV if chest pain not relieved by NTG SL. Begin at 20 mcg/min. may titrate to chest pain.
14. Morphine 4 mg IVP STAT

VITAL SIGNS Time: 1115	
Blood pressure	170/88
Heart rate	102
Respirations	22
Temperature	98 F
Pulse oximetry	88 %

Place the items in the box below in the appropriate column

Order	Implement now	Complete within 1 hour	Complete by end of shift	Complete within 24 hours
Admit to coronary care unit				
Nitroglycerin SL				
Oxygen via nasal cannula				
Continuous cardiac monitor				
Continuous pulse oximetry				
EKG				
2-D echo				
NPO				
Cardiology consult				
Bedrest				
Vital signs				
Aspirin 325 mg				
Initial assessment				
Nitroglycerin infusion				
Morphine				

Fill in the blank on ways this patient can begin a healthy lifestyle regime.

Diet	
Activity	
Smoking	
Alcohol consumption	
Weight	
Wellness checkups	
Stress	
other	

Choose from the list below, the members that would be anticipated to be on this patients interdisciplinary team. Mark an X for those that should be on the team

Healthcare personnel	Team
Primary physician	
Nurse	
Cardiologist	
Respiratory therapist	
Dietician	
Nutritionist	
Diabetic educator	
Patient care technician	
Case manager	
Pharmacist	
Physical therapist	
Occupational therapist	
Nuclear medication technician	
Charge nurse	

Vital signs/ time: 1200

B/P: 148/84. HR: 92. RR: 20. POX: 93%

Place the data in the appropriate box

	Improved	Declined	No change
B/P 148/84			
HR 92			
RR 20			
POX 93%			

Explain in the box below, why the doctor set the oxygenation parameters at 88 – 92 %

CVA SCENERIO

1. You are caring for a patient that has been admitted for a right-sided CVA. You assess your patient. You notice when the patient extends both arms, palms up, the left arm drops downward while the right arm remains in the initial position. Using the table below, what is this result called? _____.

Pronator drift
Expressive aphasia
Ptosis
Anisocoria
Babinski

2. The patient attempts to ask for a drink of water but he is unable to speak. Using the table above, what is the patient's issue? _____

3. Using your pen light, you assess the patient's pupils. You notice that one pupil is 3 mm smaller than the other. Using the table above, what is this condition called? _____.

4. The doctor comes in while you are assessing the patient. The doctor strokes the lateral side of the bottom of the patients foot. The large toe moves upward and the toes fan out. Using the table above, what is this reflex test called? _____. Is this response considered negative or positive? _____.

5. You are assessing if your patient has a facial droop. Before you can ask your patient to smile, you notice one of the patient's eye lids is half closed while the other eye lid is appropriately up. Using the table above, what is this condition? _____.

Diabetes mellites next-gen scenario

62 year-old male brought in by ambulance (BIBA). Patient had been participating in a local senior walking marathon when he began to experience sudden onset of fatigue accompanied by slurred speech. Past medical history (PMH): Total right knee replacement, diabetes type II, and ex-smoker.

List in order which of the following should be implemented <u>immediately</u>. Mark only those that apply.

X-ray	
Neurological assessment	
MRI	
Vital signs	
Insert and IV	
Fingerstick	
CT scan	
Ultrasound	

Vital signs/Time: 1330	
Blood pressure	150/92
Heart rate	110
Respirations	22
Temperature	97.4 F
Pulse oximetry	93 %

NURSE NOTE: Patient drowsy but arousable with verbal stimuli. Speech slurred. PERRLA. Grasp equal bilateral. Able to move all extremities (MAE). Heart rate tachycardia. Lungs CTA. Abdomen soft, non-tender, with positive bowel sounds. Hesitancy when voiding. Diaphoretic and pale. Labs drawn and sent. IV initiated. Patient placed on cardiac monitor. Continuous pulse oximetry in progress.

Laboratory results		Normal level
Fingerstick	38 mg/dL	70 -99 mg/dL
hemoglobin	15 g/dL	14 – 17 g/dL
Sodium	126 mEq/L	135 – 145 mEq/L
Potassium	3.3 mEq/L	3.5 – 5.2 mEq/L
BUN	26	6 – 24 mg/dL
Creatinine	2.1	0.7 – 1.2 mg/dL
Glucose	35 mg/dL	70 – 99 mg/dL

Based on the above results, which of the following are appropriate interventions

INTERVENTION	
D50 IVP stat	
IVF of 0.9 NS at 75 ml/hr.	
Recheck fingerstick in 2 hours	
Potassium 10 mEq po	
IVF of D5NS at 50 ml/hr.	
Recheck labs in 2 hours	
Potassium 10 mEq IV X 2	
Recheck fingerstick in 30 min.	
Recheck labs in am	
4 oz. orange juice & 4 oz. milk	

Which of the following is the anticipated diagnosis

Cerebral vascular accident (CVA)	
Hypoglycemia	
Bell's palsy	
hypertension	
dehydration	

Choose which of the following are signs of this diagnosis

Weakness	
Sweating	
Thirsty	
Seizure	
Bradycardia	

Tremors	
Slurred speech	
Irregular pupils	

List patient data that is missing from the initial assessment

1.

2.

3.

4.

Choose which of the following would be appropriate patient teaching

Carry glucose tablets	
Eat a high protein diet before exercise	
Hold insulin when exercising	
1 unit of insulin reduces bs by 30 – 50 mg/dL	
Exercise increases blood sugar levels	
Never exercise if blood glucose is low	
Use a glucometer to monitor blood sugar levels	

Based on the patient's lack of knowledge, choose which of the following should be consulted.

Dietician	
Endocrinologist	
Diabetic educator	
Physical medicine physician	
neurologist	

HEMATOLOGY SCENERIO

1. Your patient has been brought in by ambulance after sustaining an industrial injury. His artery was severed and he has lost a lot of blood. From the table below, what blood type would you give emergently without cross-matching? _____.

1. Type B and type O
2. Type AB, A, B, and O
3. Type B and O
4. Only type O

2. Which of the blood types above is considered the universal donor?

3. Which of the blood types above is considered the universal recipient?

4. After the patient is taken to surgery, you notice his laboratory results reflect the following blood type for your patient, type **B+**.

The doctor orders 4 units of packed-red blood cells (PRBC) to be transfused. You realize the patient's intravenous catheter (IV) has infiltrated. You need to start an IV in order to transfuse the PRBC. What size IV needle will you use in order to transfuse? (choose the most preferred size). _____

1. 22 gauge
2. 23 gauge
3. 14 gauge
4. 18 gauge

5. What IV fluids will you use to prime and flush the transfusion? _____

a. D5W
b. D10W
c. LR
d. ½ NS

e. D5NS
f. NS
g. ¼ NS

PARKINSON'S next-gen DISEASE

A 73 year-old man is admitted with a diagnosis of Parkinson's disease. Choose from the following, which, if any, are used to diagnose Parkinson's disease.

	Used to diagnose P.D.
EMG & NCV	
Anti-acetylcholine receptor antibody test	
PMH & Symptoms	
MRI	

The nurse knows there are classical symptoms of Parkinson's disease, known as the triad of P.D. Choose from the list below those symptoms.

	Symptom of Parkinson's disease
Rigidity	
Ptosis	
Lhermitte's sign	
Bradykinesia	
Tremors at rest	
Muscle wasting	
Restless leg syndrome	

Which of the following is the initial sign of Parkinson's disease

	Initial sign
Cognitive wheel rigidity	
Festination (shuffling gait)	
Pill rolling	
Masked face	

The doctor orders diphenhydramine (Benadryl) for the Parkinson's disease patient. You anticipate this medication is ordered to:

	Answer
Control allergies	
Manage tremors	
Assist to sleep	
Rash	

As a nurse, you recognize nutrition management is important. Choose which of the following is not a good nutritional choice for the patient taking Levodopa.

	Answer
Provide adequate roughage	
Provide fortified cereals	
Provide cut food into small bite size pieces	
Provide 6 small meals daily	

Which of the following does not result in drug(s) induced Parkinson's disease.

	Answer
Methyldopa	
Propranolol	
Lithium	
Haloperidol	
chlorpromazine	

The doctor discusses a deep-brain stimulator (DBS). Choose which of the following area that is not considered for electrode placement.

	Answer
Thalamus	
Lateral Corticospinal tract	
Subthalmic nucleus	
Globus pallidus	

CRITICAL THINKING SCENERIO EXERCISE 1

A 68 year old man was brought in by ambulance (BIBA) to the emergency room (ER). The patient was found down on a side walk by a jogger. The patient was unconscious when the emergency medical services (EMS) arrived but regained consciousness shortly afterward.

A 5.08 centimeter (2 inch) laceration to the right forehead was noted. The patient is now alert and oriented. A plastic surgery consult is ordered to evaluate and treat the facial laceration.

    A. What do you believe the patient's diagnosis may be?

Could the patient have been mugged? Could the patient have had a transient ischemic attack (TIA) or a cerebral vascular accident (CVA)? Could the patient have vertigo and lost his balance? Could any of the above be a cause for this patient's condition? Using your knowledge and skills, what other possible diagnoses could this patient have?

    B. What do you anticipate the doctor will order?

You begin to assess the patient. Pupils are equally reactive to light and accommodation (PERRLA). You have the patient place both palms facing upward and raise both arms up. The patient is asked to keep the arms up to the count of 10. Both arms remain up with no drift (downward movement). You ask the patient to hold his right leg up to the count of 5. He is able to do this without difficulty. You ask him to relax his right leg and now lift his left leg up to the count of 5. He is able to do this without difficulty. You ask him to relax his left leg. You grasp both hands and ask the patient to squeeze simultaneously. His grasps are equal and strong. You place your hands in front of the patients toes and ask the patient to pull his toes toward himself while you provide resistance. He does this without difficulty. You place your hands on the bottom of the patient's feet and ask him to push on your hands as if pushing on the gas pedal of a car. He does this without any difficulty.

C. Based on this assessment, can you rule out (R/O) the patient did not have a TIA or CVA?

You ask the patient if he has ever had a seizure. The patient asks, "What is a seizure?" Based on the patient's response, can you R/O the patient had a seizure?

The patient requests to use the bathroom. You assist the patient off the gurney. You follow the patient closely and notice he has a shuffling gait. You remember from nursing school that a shuffling gait is a symptom of Parkinson's disease. Based on this new finding, can you determine this patient has Parkinson's disease?

The doctor ordered a CT scan and blood tests. The CT scan result shows negative for a CVA. The blood work is within normal limit (WNL) with the exception of the HgA1C of 9.4 and a glucose level of 380.

You question the patient further regarding his health history and discover the patient is a diabetic II. He has a history of neuropathy and his feet are numb. The patient admits to having fallen in the past due to his inability to feel the ground under his feet.

After reviewing all the data, were you able to use your knowledge and skills to determine the patient's true diagnosis? Student nurses must learn to use critical thinking to plan the patient's care and provide patient safety.

CRITICAL THINKING SCENARIO EXERCISE 2

Nursing students are always hearing the term " critical thinking". This skill develops with a good knowledge foundation and the ability to collect data and analyze that data. An example is given below.

The police bring an elderly woman into the emergency room. The woman is dressed in a tee-shirt and underwear. No bra, pants, or shoes. The woman is confused and cannot offer any information. She doesn't even know her name. The police said a home owner had called when this elderly woman attempted unsuccessfully to enter the home via a locked front door.

The woman appears mid-eighties, slightly pale. Vital signs as follows: BP 184/92, HR 88, RR 20, t 100.4. Pulse oximetry (PO) 94%.

Based on these findings, can we determine the patient's diagnosis?

Alzheimer's? Dementia? Cerebral vascular accident (CVA)? Brain tumor? Meningitis?

What would you anticipate the doctor to order?

A computerized tomography (CT) scan? Magnetic Resonance imaging (MRI), chest X-ray, blood work, psychology consult?

The doctor orders a CT scan and blood work, along with an urinalysis.

The CT scan is negative for a CVA or tumor. The CT scan is negative for atrophy which would confirm Alzheimer's.

The WBC count is elevated.

The urinalysis is positive for 2+ bacteria.

Dementia cannot be ruled out without the patient's past medical history and a cognitive function test.

Meningitis can be confirmed with a lumbar punction, however; the patient does not present with the usual symptoms of meningitis. High temperatures, severe headache, a stiff neck, and drowsiness.

The urinalysis shows bacteria 2+, which means a urinary tract infection.

Using critical thinking, we can determine this patient most likely has a urinary tract infection. Often an elderly woman with a urinary tract infection becomes confused. The infection causes a reaction in the body. The inflammation results in stress which can result in confusion.

It is important for nursing students to know the classic symptoms of diseases and the how to confirm the diagnosis of those diseases. As seen with this example, many symptoms can make it difficult to diagnose a specific disease. Thus, the reason, assessments and data collection are the key.

CRITICAL THINKING SCENERIO EXERCISE 3

A male patient brought in by ambulance (BIBA) was found down in the men's bathroom of a local restaurant. The patient was drowsy on arrival. Skin is cool and clammy.

Based on the information you currently know, what can you anticipate to be the underlying cause that resulted in this patient being found down?

Could it have been a myocardial infarction (MI) ? A cerebral vascular accident (CVA) ? Choking on food?

The answer is yes to all the potential diagnoses but more data is required.

On your initial assessment, the patient's vital signs are 172/94 – HR 58- RR 12- 96.2F.

Based on your initial assessment and vital signs findings, can any of the possible diagnoses be ruled out?

The patient is not coughing which may indicate aspiration of food. This may rule out aspiration but a CX-ray should be ordered by the doctor to confirm aspiration has not occurred.

The patient is not guarding his chest or complaining of chest pain. This may rule out a myocardial infarction. However, a diabetic patient may not experience the typical signs and symptoms of an MI. Diabetics have been known to have "silent MIs". The doctor should order an electrocardiogram (EKG) and troponin levels. An EKG can show ischemia or cardiac injury. Troponin levels above 0.04 indicate cardiac injury.

A neurological assessment yields no abnormalities. This may rule out (R/O) a cerebral vascular accident (CVA), however; the doctor should order a CT scan of the brain to r/o CVA.

What can be the cause of the low respirations? What additional data would you collect?

Did the patient smoke? An exacerbation of emphysema could result in difficulty in breathing (DIB). The CXR would show hyperinflated lungs if this were the cause.

Does the patient have a history of asthma? An asthmatic patient who fails to follow a prescribed medication regime or has exposure to an allergen, can result in airway obstruction or increased mucus rendering breathing difficulties. However; would the respiratory rate be normal if this occurred?

The CT scan is negative. This r/o the diagnosis of a CVA.

The EKG is normal. Troponin levels are less than 0.04 nanograms per milliliter (ng/mL). This r/o the diagnosis of MI.

The CXR shows no abnormalities. This can r/o emphysema.

Using what data is available, what could have caused this patient to have a syncopal episode? Often the nurse must analyze all the data available to ensure the patient receives the appropriate care.

Reviewing the information: He was found down in a restaurant. Did he have any allergies? Did he consume alcohol? The doctor orders a blood alcohol test.

The laboratory reports that the blood alcohol level is 0.28g/100mL.

Based on the data, you can determine the patient has alcohol poisoning. Signs of alcohol poisoning are: slow respirations, low temperature, drowsiness, and clammy skin. The laboratory test confirms this diagnosis.

What additional information should the nurse know regarding patients that consume alcohol? What medications may the patient be taking. Some medications when consumed along with alcohol can cause additional stress on the liver. This can make affect the liver's ability to process the medications rendering them less effective and may result in liver damage.

A patient with a high alcohol level should be monitored for withdrawal symptoms. Delirium tremens may appear. The presence of agitation, changes in mental status, or deliriums must be monitored and reported. Often sedation must be administered to ease the patient through the withdrawal period. There are several alcohol assessment tools. Each institute determines which tool will be used.

It should also be noted that one can not assume the patient has a disease process that caused the current health problem. The patient should have been tested for drugs of abuse (DOA). A thorough physical assessment to ensure the patient was not assaulted.

Although time will often help to determine the underlying cause, often patients do not have time on their side. The hypoglycemic patient, if not given a dose of glucose, could die. If the patient is a known diabetic, it is prudent to give dextrose to ensure the patient is not hypoglycemic.

If a drug overdose is suspected, the patient should be given a drug reversal agent based on the anticipated drug type consumed.

Knowledge is necessary when caring for patients.

The following pages are answers to the assignments, worksheets, next-gen and critical thinking scenarios. Some worksheets cannot be answered due to the nature of their content. Such as a community windshield survey or worksheets based on patient assignments. Answers are included when applicable.

ABDOMINAL SYSTEM 1 answers

1. Define the following

Glycogenolysis	Carbohydrates in the form of glycogen is stored in the liver which is broken down when needed by the body
glycogenesis	The process of glycogen synthesized from glucose
Glyconeogenesis	The process of synthesizing new glucose from non-carbohydrate substances (proteins & fats)

2. Give a brief explanation of the liver's relationship in the following.

Fats	When the body is low on glucose, the liver can convert stored fats into glycerol and fat for energy
Proteins	Protein is used to repair body tissue. Amino acids are converted into protein by the liver when needed. The liver also makes albumin
Bilirubin	When the body breaks down red blood cells, the bilirubin is released. The liver changes bilirubin into bile.
Hormones	The liver is the site where hormones are metabolized.
Vitamins	Vitamins are metabolized and stored in the liver
Clotting	Vitamin K plays a role in blood clotting and can only be absorbed with bile which is produced by the liver

3. What is cirrhosis? Cirrhosis is fibrosis (scarring) of the liver. This scarring prevents the liver from working adequately.

4. List two causes of cirrhosis.

   a. excessive alcohol consumption
   b. hepatitis B, hepatitis C
   c. Fatty liver

5. Explain what is encephalopathy and its relationship to liver failure. Encephalopathy is a neurological abnormality that occurs when there is an accumulation of neuro toxins in the brain. Encephalopathy occurs when high levels of ammonia accumulate in the body due to liver damage.

ACID-BASE BALANCE 1 answers

1. Lists three types of patients that are at risk for an acid-base imbalance.
   a. patients with excessive vomiting
   b. COPD patients
   c. Renal failure

2. What is the role of pH in acid-base balance? The pH measures the concentration of hydrogen ions in the blood and determines alkalosis or acidosis.

3. How is the pH measured? The pH is measured (in the body) using a scale measuring hydrogen ions in the blood.

4. Explain why arterial blood must be used instead of venous blood when assessing the acid-base status. Arterial blood is able to measure oxygenated blood whereas, venous blood is unoxygenated.

5. Define the following and their values.

pH	A way to measure acidity or alkalosis in a solution. 7.35 – 7.45
PaCO2	Partial pressure of carbon dioxide. This level determines the amount of carbon dioxide in the blood. 35 – 45 mm Hg
PaO2	Partial pressure of oxygen. This level measures the amount of oxygen in the blood. 75 – 100 mm Hg
HCO3	Bicarbonate is a negatively charged electrolyte that assists the body to balance the pH. 22 – 28 mEq/L
SaO2	This represents the saturation of oxygen in arterial blood. 95 – 100%
Base Excess (BE)	Is a value representing the amount of base or acid needed to balance the pH

6. What is a chemical buffer system? A system that attempts to maintain the constant pH balance of the blood.

7. What is meant by compensation? The body's attempt to maintain the acid-base balance in the body through the use of the respiratory or renal system.

8. Explain the role of the lungs and the kidneys in maintaining acid-base imbalance.

The lungs alter ventilation in efforts to keep the pH within normal parameters. If the pH is low (acidic) the respiratory rate will increase to "blow off" CO_2. If the pH is high, the respiratory rate may lower in efforts to increase CO_2 levels and decrease the alkalosis.
The kidneys produce Bicarb in efforts to reduce acidity of the blood. The production of Bicarb may be reduced in the pH reflects alkalosis.

ALLERGY WORKSHEET ANSWERS

1. What symptoms may be observed in common seasonal allergies? Runny nose, watery eyes, sneezing, and coughing

2. Briefly explain why allergies affect some people while other people are unaffected. It is believed that the person's immunity and genetics play a role in the allergic response.

3. What is it called when someone has a lethal allergic reaction? An anaphylactic reaction or anaphylactic shock.

4. Is contact dermatitis an allergy? Explain your response. It may be an allergic reaction. If the person has an allergy to detergent, the skin may react when in contact with detergent.

5. Describe symptoms that may present in contact dermatitis. . Itching, redness, and rash may occur when exposed to an allergen, such as detergent.

6. Is asthma considered an allergy? Explain your response. Asthma can be an allergy as a trigger may cause an asthmatic episode. However, asthma may be triggered by other things, such cold air or exercise.

7. Describe symptoms that may present in asthma. Exercised or cold induced asthma may cause coughing and bronchial spasms. Asthma from an allergy can result in increased mucus production, constriction of the bronchial tubes, and restrictive oxygen intake.

ASSESSMENT 1 answers

Match the following to its correct definition.

Topic	definition
1. Inspection	a. Therapeutic touch of the human body to obtain information
2. Palpitation	b. Hitting an object against another resulting in vibrations to elicit sounds
3. Percussion	c. Use of vision and sense of smell to gather data

1. ___c___   2. ___a___   3. ___b___

2. What is the purpose of a nursing assessment? **To gather information regarding the patient's health and current health concerns.**

3. What is the difference between an initial nursing assessment and a shift assessment? **The initial assessment is completed on admission and includes a very thorough head-to-toe assessment of the patient. A shift assessment is more focused on the patient's health issue.**

4. Which of the assessment skills in the box above would be used to assess a skin rash? **Inspection**

5. Which of the assessment skills in the box above would be used to assess pulses? **Palpation**

6. Which of the assessment skills in the box above would be used to assess a distended abdomen? **Percussion**

7. Which of the assessment skills in the box above would be used to assess a pressure ulcer? **Inspection**

8. What is auscultation? **Listening to sounds of the body with the use of a stethoscope.**

9. Which organ would you use the diaphragm and the bell of your stethoscope to auscultate? **The diaphragm is used to auscultate the lungs, the heart, and gastrointestinal sounds. The bell is used to auscultate sounds such as heart murmurs.**

10. Which skill would be first when assessing respirations, auscultation, or inspection? **The nurse should first assess respiratory effort. The nurse should assess if the use of accessory**

muscles are in use. Then the nurse should auscultated for wheezes, rhonchi, crackles, or rales.

11. Explain a problem that may occur when palpating a pulse. **The pulse may be weak and difficult to palpate. The pulse may be difficult to find, such as the popliteal or posterior tibial pulse.**

12. Which skills may be involved to assess the capillary refill. **The nurse must compress the nail bed or finger/toe for 10 seconds (palpation). The pressure results in pallor. When the pressure is released, the color should return in less than 3 seconds.**

BASIC NURSING KNOWLEDGE 1 answers

1. List the areas that intramuscular injections may be administered.

   Deltoid, vastus lateralis, ventrogluteal, and dorsogluteal muscles

2. List the areas that a subcutaneous injection may be administered.

   Arms, legs, or abdomen.

3. List the veins that an intravenous infusion catheter may be inserted. List which veins you would access first.

   First: dorsal metacarpal (the hand)
   Second: Cephalic, basilic,
   Third: antecubital

4. What is a saline lock? **A tube placed within the vein capped but will allow access if needed to instill medication or intravenous fluids.**

5. What is a continuous infusion? **A fluid infused into the blood stream via an intracatheter over a longer duration of time.**

6. What does incompatibility refer to when discussing intravenous infusions? **An undesirable reaction when two solutions or drugs are mixed which may cause unsafe therapeutic results**.

7. What is an IV bolus? **A prescribed amount of fluid given in a short amount of time.**

8. When would a bolus be used? **When the status of the patient requires it. An example, if the patient's glucose is very low, an IV bolus of dextrose would be given rapidly. If the patient's blood pressure is low, a fluid bolus would be given rapidly.**

BLOOD TRANSFUSION WORKSHEET answers

1. List the four blood types: ___A_____, ___B_____, ____AB_____, _____O_____.

2. Does not have antigens	2a. O-	
3. Type A + may receive these blood types	3a. A-, A+, O+, O-	Using your answers from above, match the following to the appropriate response
4. Type B+ may receive these blood types	4a. B+, B-, O+, O-	
5. Type AB+ may receive these blood types	5a. A+, A-, B+, B-, AB+, AB-, O+, O-	
6. Type AB- may receive these blood types	6a. A-, B-, O-	
7. Type O + may receive these blood types	7a. O+, O-	
8. Type O – may receive these blood types	8a. O-	
9. Type considered the universal donor	9a. O-	
10. Is considered the universal recipient	10a. AB+	
11. Type A – may receive these blood types	11a. A+, A-, O-	
12. Type B- may receive these blood types	12a. B-, O-	

A. What is the maximum duration red blood cells can be transfused? _____4 HOURS_____.
B. What is the duration fresh frozen plasma can be transfused? _____30 minutes_____.
C. What is the duration platelets can be transfused? _____1 hour_____.

CARDIAC 1 answers

1. Define the following and list their role in caring for a cardiac patient

Echocardiogram	An ultrasound of the heart used to diagnose heart disease
Stress test	A monitored test to assess the functioning of the heart during physical activity
Troponin	A cardiac cell protein that leaks into the blood stream when the heart muscle is damaged
Myoglobin	A striated muscle protein
Cholesterol	A fat produced in the liver
HDL	A high-density lipoprotein known as the "good" cholesterol
LDL	A low-density lipoprotein known as the "bad" cholesterol
Triglycerides	Most common type of fat in the body. It enters the body via food consumption

2. Define the difference between the following

ANGINA	MYOCARDIAL INFARCTION
Chest pain that improves with rest **Fatigue** **Weakness** **Short of breath**	Chest pain not relieved with rest Pain travels from left arm to neck, or jaw Diaphoretic Nausea Vomiting Abnormal heart rate

	Anxiety

3. What is heart failure? **When the heart is unable to effectively pump enough blood to meet the body's requirements.**

CARDIAC 2 answers

1. List the difference between right ventricular and left ventricular heart failure.

Left ventricular heart failure	Right ventricle heart failure
Shortness of breath.	**Jugular vein distention**
Rales	**Pulmonary hypertension**
Decreased breath sounds	**Ascites**
Weight gain.	**Crackles**
Cyanosis.	**Hypotension**
Chronic cough	**Peripheral edema**

2. Which cardiac ventricle pumps blood into the periphery? **Left ventricle**

3. Which cardiac ventricle pumps blood to the lungs? **Right ventricle**

4. When would JVD be observed? **When blood backs up in the superior vena cava in right sided heart failure**

5. When would peripheral edema be observed? **In congestive heart failure, the pumping strength of heart is weakened resulting in blood back up in the more distal extremities (legs) resulting in edema.**

6. List the four valves of the heart.

Mitral valve
Tricuspid valve
Aortic valve

Pulmonary valve

7. Define the following

Cardiac output (CO)	**The amount of blood pumped by the heart per minute**
Stroke volume	**The amount of blood pumped out of the heart's left ventricle with each cardiac contraction**

CARDIAC 3 answers

1. List signs and symptoms a patient with congested heart failure may demonstrate.

Fatigue, short of breath, chronic cough, peripheral edema, and weight gain

2. List the different causes of heart failure.

Modifiable	Nonmodifiable
Diet	Gender
Exercise	Race
Stop smoking	Family history
Reduce stress	age
Limit alcohol consumption	

3. What other health care team members should be included in the heart failure patient's care and their role?

Healthcare team member	Role in the patient's care
Cardiologist	Manage cardiac care

Nurse Respiratory therapist Case manager pharmacist dietician	Pt. teaching. Implement cardiac regime Monitor need for supplemental oxygen Manage home needs (equipment, healthcare staff) Provide medications. Provide healthy diet

4. Patient teaching is important. Explain what patient education, you as the nurse, would give the heart failure patient.

Education	Rationale
Monitor weight daily Activity Medications Diet symptoms	Weight gain is a sign the heart may be worsening and the doctor should be notified. Exercise to improve heart health The patient should be educated on the each medication The patient should be instructed on what food to avoid. Low fat, low sodium. The patient should be educated on what symptoms to monitor for and when to notify the doctor.

CARDIAC 4 answers

1. Describe techniques for auscultating your patient's heart sounds. **Explain to the patient what you will be doing. Listen to the 4 valves and Erb's point using the diaphragm of the stethoscope. Using the bell, auscultate for murmurs**

2. What are considered normal heart sounds? **A lub dub can be heard from the sound of the closing of the atrioventricular valves.**

3. What are considered abnormal heart sounds? **Murmurs or rubbing.**

4. What is a murmur? **An abnormal flowing of blood through the heart valves**

5. List two issues that would cause a murmur. **Heart valve disease, anemia, infection, and anxiety or stress.**

6. Your patient is grossly obese. His weight makes it difficult to hear heart sounds. Is there anything that can be done to assist to hear the heart sounds? Explain your answer. **Turn the patient onto his left side. This will bring the heart closer to the chest wall making it easier to auscultate.**

7. What valves make the S1 heart sound? **The closure of the atrioventricular valves (tricuspid and mitral).**

8. What valves make the S2 heart sound? **The closure of the semilunar valves (aortic and pulmonary)**

9. Should the nurse use the diaphragm or bell of the stethoscope to auscultate heart sounds? Explain your response. **Both. The diaphragm to auscultate to high-frequency heart sounds and the bell of the stethoscope to auscultate for low-frequency sounds (murmurs).**

10. Where would you auscultate the apical pulse? **At the 5th intercostal space to the left of the midclavicular line**

11. While auscultating your patient's heart, you note the heart rhythm is irregular with a varying rate. What rhythm would you anticipate this patient to be diagnosed with? Explain your response. **Atrial fibrillation because atrial fibrillation is an irregular heart rhythm.**

12. While auscultating your patient's heart, you hear a strange rubbing sound. Since you know the heart normally makes a S1 and S2 sound, should you be concerned? Explain your response.

This could be a pericardial rub which may indicate a pericardial effusion. This should be reported immediately to the doctor.

CARDIAC 5 answers

1. List five symptoms a patient in heart failure may demonstrate on admission.

Short of breath
fatigue
weakness
Peripheral edema
Chronic cough

2. How can heart failure affect activities of daily living? The patient may have to plan ahead. Activities may cause shortness of breath. So activities may need to be spaced out. Choosing priorities.

List three causes of heart failure.
Coronary artery disease
hypertension
endocarditis

3. List signs or symptoms of deteriorating heart failure.

Weight gain of 2 or more pounds in one day.
Increased edema in lower extremities
Short of breath at rest

4. What patient education should be discussed with a patient that has been newly diagnosed with heart failure? Prescribed medication, activities, weight monitoring, cardiac diet, and what symptoms to monitor.

5. Why is it important for the diagnosed cardiac patient to follow a low sodium diet? To prevent the retention of fluids which may cause worsening symptoms.

6. What is the purpose of obtaining a daily weight in the patient with a history of heart failure? Weight gain is an indicator of fluid retention. Two or more pounds gained in a 24 hour period should be reported to the doctor.

CARDIAC 6 answer

Match the following

Cardiac drug	
1 Ace inhibitor	d. Lowers blood pressure and decreases heart rate
2 Angiotensin receptor blocker (ARB)	e. Rids the body of excess fluid. Decreases swelling.
3 Beta blocker	f. Alters hormones that may cause damage to the heart
4. diuretic	d. lowers blood pressure and decreases the work load of the heart
5. aldosterone antagonist	e. lowers heart rate. Helps the heart pump more efficiently
6. antiarrhythmic	f. lowers blood pressure and decreases the work load of the heart

1__D_____ 2. __F_____ 3. ___A____ 4. ___B_____ 5. __C_____ 6. ____E____

2. Why should patients on cardiac medications be made aware of over-the-counter (OTC) drug interaction? Some over-the-counter medications increase blood pressure

3. Explain the relationship between stress and heart failure. Stress can increase blood pressure. It can also cause inflammation.

4. Explain how smoking affects the heart. Nicotine can constrict blood vessels resulting in a reduction of blood flowing to the heart.

5. What is an echocardiogram? An ultrasound of the heart to determine the function of the heart

6. What information can be obtained from an echocardiogram? If the heart valves are functioning properly

7. What is an ejection fraction? It is the amount of blood pumped from the heart during each heartbeat.

8. What is a normal ejection fraction? Greater than 40 percent

9. What is an electrocardiogram? A test that determines the electrical signals of the heart

10. What does idiopathic mean? A condition that occurs spontaneously from an unknown cause.

Conversion practice worksheet answers

1. 2 g = __2000__ mg
2. 1 mg = __1000__ mcg
3. 25,000 mcg = __25__ mg
4. 3 L = __3000__ mL
5. 125 mcg = __0.125__ mg
6. 275 mL = __0.275__ L
7. 2.5 L = __2500__ mL
8. 3 tsp = __1__ T
9. 8 oz. = __240__ mL
10. ½ gallon = __64__ oz.
11. 0.5 mg = __500__ mcg

12. 2.65000 mg =   __0.00265_____ g

13. 30 oz. =   ___900_____ mL

14. 4 oz. =   ___0.5_____ C

15. 15 oz. =   ____30_____ T

16. 10 mL =   _____2_____ tsp

CRITICAL CARE answers

1. List examples of cardiac emergencies.

A myocardial infarction
A cardiac arrest
Chest pain
Pericardial tamponade
pericarditis
Pulseless electrical activity
Ventricular tachycardia
Ventricular fibrillation

2. List those who would be needed at the bedside of a code blue and their role

Assigned nurse to notify the MD of the current situation and patient's past medical history	Physician to run the code
Respiratory therapist to apply oxygen, assist with suctioning, and provide supplemental oxygen equipment (vent)	2 persons to perform CPR. May be nursing assistance, patient care tech, or nurses
Medication administration nurse	Nurse to record the code
Runner for supplies. Can be a nurse, nursing assistant, or patient care tech.	Someone to notify the family or stay with the family. Can be charge nurse or nurse

3. List at least two certifications a nurse working in a critical care area, such as ER, OR, ICU, may require
   a. Basic life support
   b. Advance cardiac life support

CRITICAL CARE 2 answers

1. List when an MRI (magnetic resonance imaging) would be contraindicated.
   When the patient has metal within the body or an implanted electrical device.

2. What must the nurse ensure prior to taking the patient for an ordered MRI?
   No medication patches are on the patient. The patient has no implanted device or metal in the body. Some hospitals require an MRI form completed to ensure the MRI is not contraindicated.

3. What is cardiac monitoring? List reasons it may be used. A device that monitors the electrical activity of the heart. To monitor a patient who may have new onset of atrial fibrillation. To monitor for cardiac irregularities. To monitor for bradycardia.

4. What is telemetry? List when telemetry may be used. A portable device that monitors the cardiac electrical activity.

5. What is hemodynamic monitoring? When would hemodynamic monitoring be used?
   A invasive procedure to monitor the functioning of the heart.

6. Define the following.

CVP	Central venous pressure is the pressure measuring the right side of the heart
PAP	Pulmonary artery pressure which measures pressures in the lungs.
PAWP	Pulmonary arterial wedge pressure is a procedure to measure the preload of the left ventricle. It is achieved by using a catheter with a balloon tip which is inflated and wedged into a pulmonary artery.
CO	The amount of blood the heart pumps in one minute.

CRITICAL CARE 3 answers

Match the type of trauma with cause of injury.

Type of trauma	Cause of trauma
1. oxygen deprivation	asphyxiation
2. electrical trauma	Wires downed
3. thermal trauma	fire
4. mechanical trauma	Motor vehicle crash (MVC)
5. electrical trauma	lighting
6. chemical trauma	toxins
7. radiation trauma	Ultra violet (UV) rays
8. thermal trauma	steam
9. mechanical trauma	fall
10. mechanical trauma	Gun shot wound (GSW)
11. chemical trauma	substances
12. oxygen deprivation	drowning
13. mechanical trauma	assault
14. thermal trauma	heat
15. radiant trauma	radioactive
16. oxygen deprivation	Carbon monoxide/dioxide inhalation
17. electrical trauma	sockets

Trauma key:

Mechanical trauma

Thermal trauma

Chemical trauma

Electrical trauma

Radiant trauma

Oxygen deprivation

CRITICAL CARE 4 answers

1. Briefly explain how acceleration-deceleration injuries occur. This injury occurs when the moving person suddenly stops but the brain within the skull continues in a forward motion and strikes the inner surface of the skull.

2. What is a coup-contrecoup? Similar to acceleration deceleration injuries, the motion stops suddenly, the brains strikes the front of the skull and the brain jolts backward and strikes the back side of the skull resulting in two injuries.

3. Explain the difference between the following fractures.

    d. Linear fracture: non-displaced break in the bone.

    e. Depressed fracture: bone displacement inward due to trauma.

    f. Basilar skull fracture: fracture of the bone(s) at the base of the skull.

4. Why must a patient with a traumatic brain injury need a cranial nerve assessment?

    A change in mental status can be indictive of a worsening or deteriorating condition.

5. Why must a patient with a traumatic brain injury be monitored for a cerebral spinal fluid leak?

    A cerebral spinal fluid leak are common when a traumatic brain injury has occurred.

6. What is parenchyma? The tissue in the brain that consisting of neurons and glial cells.

Briefly define each of the following and their location

7. Brain tissue: Tissue of the brain that allows communication throughout the body via electrical signals. Located within the cranium.

8. Pia matter: connective tissue that surrounds the brain. Assists to provide cerebrospinal fluid to the brain.

9. Meninges: membranes (3- dura, arachnoid, and pia mater) that cover the brain and spinal cord. The meninges allow circulation, and protect the brain.

10. Cerebrum: The cerebrum is the largest part of the brain. Divided into two hemispheres. Controls speech, thought processes, and emotions.

11. Cerebellum: The structure located near the brain stem that provides balance and movements.

12. Brain stem: Located at the base of the brain, the brain stem connects the cerebrum and diencephalon with the spinal cord.

CVA SCENERIO answers

1. You are caring for a patient that has been admitted for a right-sided CVA. You assess your patient. You notice when the patient extends both arms, palms up, the left arm drops downward while the right arm remains in the initial position. Using the table below, what is this result called? ___pronator drift_____ .

Pronator drift
Expressive aphasia
Ptosis
Anisocoria
Babinski

2. The patient attempts to ask for a drink of water but he is unable to speak. Using the table above, what is the patient's issue? _____expressive aphasia_____

3. Using your pen light, you assess the patient's pupils. You notice that one pupil is 3 mm smaller than the other. Using the table above, what is this condition called? __anisocoria_____ .

4. The doctor comes in while you are assessing the patient. The doctor strokes the lateral side of the bottom of the patients foot. The large toe moves upward and the toes fan out. Using the table above, what is this reflex test called? _____Babinski_____ . Is this response considered negative or positive? __positive_____ .

5. You are assessing if your patient has a facial droop. Before you can ask your patient to smile, you notice one of the patient's eye lids is half closed while the other eye lid is appropriately up. Using the table above, what is this condition? __ptosis_____ .

DEATH AND DYING 1 answers

1. List three people that the family of your dying patient may request to see.

    a. clergy
    b. family
    c. friends

2. Your patient's widow asks, "Did my husband have a lot of pain before he died?" What is your response if you were unable to make the patient completely comfortable. Explain your response.

    You would not want the family to know the patient suffered during the dying process. You can explain you made the patient as comfortable as possible.

3. Your dying patient is listed as an organ donor. What would you need to do or contact?
   The organ procurement organization in your area.

4. List two things you, as the nurse, can do for yourself to assist in dealing with the grief from caring for your dying patient?

    a. Talk to clergy
    b. Talk to friend or fellow nurse

5. What is comfort care? The process of providing the patient the most comfortable support possible. This may include pain control, emotional and spiritual support.

6. What is euthanasia? The process of ending a person's life to prevent suffering.

7. Is euthanasia legal? If so, list where and when is it legal? Euthanasia has limited legality. It is in the Netherlands, Belgium, Luxemburg, Colombia, Canada, Victoria, and western Australia and only several states in the United States.

8. What are the five stages of grief as per the Kubler-Ross model. Denial, anger, bargaining, depression, and acceptance.

9. Does a dying patient go through the five stages of grief in order? Explain your answer. The patient may not go through the five stages in order. The emotions may change resulting in a change in which stage the patient may be in at the time.

DELEGATION & LICENSURE answers

1. List the relationship between supervision and delegation. Briefly explain each role.
The supervisor must continue to provide supervision and guidance to the delegate. The delegate is required to follow the instructions given by the supervisor and complete the task assigned.

2. List the five factors that must be met before a nurse may delegate a task. Choose the task. Ensure to choose the right person for the task. Provide clear instructions (task, time, etc.), Assign the task. Monitor the progress of the assigned task.

3. Once a task is delegated, can that task be re-delegate? Explain your response. No. A delegated task must be completed by the person assigned the tasks.

4. Must all delegated tasks be supervised? Explain your response. Yes, all delegated tasks must be supervised. The registered nurse is accountable for all tasks assigned.

5. List the nursing personnel that are allowed to delegate. Explain which staff cannot delegate and the reason why. The registered nurse and licensed practical nurse can assign the patient care technician or nursing assistant a task. The licensed practical nurse cannot assign a registered nurse a task. A registered nurse can assign the licensed practical nurse a task.

6. Explain what should be done if you are assigned a task that you have not been trained to perform? Notify the charge nurse or the unit manager.

7. Each state determines the scope of practice of a nurse. What other limitations may be imposed and by what those limitations are imposed by. The organization may have protocols and procedures in their rules of the organization that limit staff.

8. Explain the differences between responsibility and accountability. Accountability is ownership of an issue. Responsibility may be a temporary task.

9. When a task is delegated, who is ultimately accountable to ensure the task was completed. The registered nurse that assigned the task.

10. What should the nurse do if the patient-care-technician is assigned a task but fails to complete the task or explain why the task was not completed? First speak to the patient-care technician to gather information why the task was not completed. If there is no appropriate reason, then the charge nurse or unit manager should be notified.

EAR 1 answers

1. What is otitis media? Infection of the middle ear

2. List three characteristics of an inner ear problem and give description of each.

vertigo	The feeling of spinning
Hearing issues	Unable to hear well
Nausea	Feeling sick with the potential intent of vomiting.

3. List an inner ear disease and briefly describe it.
   Meniere disease. It is caused by fluid in the inner ear chambers resulting in vertigo, nausea, vomiting, loss of hearing, and ringing in the ears.

4. What is an acoustic neuroma? A tumor that grows on the main nerve of the inner ear. It is noncancerous.

5. What is a benign paroxysmal vertigo and when does it occur? Benign paroxysmal vertigo is a feeling of dizziness, or unsteadiness when moving.

6. What safety issue may occur when a patient has an inner or middle ear infection. Explain your answer. Falling is of great concern due to dizziness.

7. List four ototoxic medications. (this answer left blank due to medication names in different areas)

8. What is a common physical finding in a patient with a middle ear infection? Pain, drainage, and the patient may complain of a sore throat
9. What is cerumen? Ear wax

EMERGENT CARE answers

1. Define what is triage and how may triage be used in healthcare. Triage is the initial assessment of a patient or casualty to determine the level of urgency for care. Triage is used in the emergency department to determine which patients should be seen first by the emergency room physician.

2. List the classification levels of triage and an example of each.

Level 1	Life threatening health issue
Level 2	Emergent. Can easily become life threatening
Level 3	Urgent but not life threatening
Level 4	Not life threatening
Level 4	Needs treatment but not is not urgent

3. List the equipment used in standard precautions. Gloves, gown, mask, and face shield. The type of standard precaution is based on the potential for splatter of bodily fluids

4. In an emergent situation. a primary survey must be performed. List the ABCDE of the survey.

A-Airway
B-breathing
C-circulation
D-disability
E-exposure

5. What is a rapid response team? List the members of the rapid response team. A rapid response team is a healthcare team that arrives at the patient's bedside when clinical deterioration occurs and provides care of the patient. The team may consist of a registered nurse, a respiratory therapist, and a nurse practitioner or a physician,

ETHICS WORKSHEET 1 answers

1. Must a child be given complete disclosure regarding their health issue or status? Explain your response. If the child is old enough to understand, yes. However; the parents or guardian must be given complete disclosure.

2. A 14-year-old girl is in active labor. Can the patient make her own decisions or must her parents be contacted to give consent? Explain your response. (This must be assessed by the instructor as each state and country has their own laws)

3. A mother and her daughter have been living on the streets. The mother is brutally stabbed. The 14-year-old daughter runs from the assailant and is hit by a bus. The girl is taken to the emergency room and pronounced brain dead. Can this patient be an organ donor? Explain the ethical dilemma involved in this case. In the United states, no. There must be a guardian, next of kin, or someone with power of attorney to give the authorization to be a donor.

4. A patient is admitted with severe arthritis. The patient states, "I don't want to live with this pain any longer." Explain the difference between chronic pain and quality of life in this patient. Chronic pain can cause depression in the patient. Chronic pain may hinder the patients quality of life. This situation should be thoroughly discussed with the patient and the patient's doctor.

5. Explain the difference between a dependent patient and an independent patient. An independent patient is a patient that provides self-care (activities of daily living) and ambulates. The dependent patient may require position changes, bathing, and feeding.

6. An 80-year-old widow is admitted with malnutrition. Your co-worker states this patient is part of the vulnerable population. Explain what is a vulnerable population and how this patient meets those criteria? A group in the community that is at risk for lack of food, financially may be below poverty level, physically not able to care for self and home, and may not have a support person or system.

7. You are assigned a patient who has a DNR on his chart. The patient is intubated. What is a DNR and how is this situation an ethical dilemma? A DNR is a do not resuscitate order. This is an ethical dilemma unless the patient's DNR was signed by a guardian or power of attorney after intubation. The patient may have also agreed to the intubation if it were a temporary situation such as if the patient had pneumonia.

8. Define justice and explain how it plays a role in healthcare. The act of being fair. Justice is implemented in healthcare by allowing anyone who needs emergent care, being seen by the doctor regardless of the ability to pay.

9. You overhear one of your coworkers say to her patient, "Dr. Purple is a quack. You should get a different doctor." Explain how this statement is slander and what repercussions can result. Slander is making statements that may damage the reputation of the person to whom the statements have been made. A lawsuit can be filed against the person who is making slanderous statements.

10. Explain the difference between neglect and abandonment. Neglect is the intentional act of failing to provide the necessary care or safety to the assigned patient. Abandonment is leaving the patient without any plan to return.

11. Explain how failure to document in the electronic medical record (EMR) can result in an ethical dilemma. Give an example. If it wasn't documented, it wasn't done. There would be no proof of any actions being completed because there is nothing in the patient's record to reflect care given. An example: A patient was given oral potassium. The potassium cause gastric distress resulting in the patient vomiting. The nurse failed to document the patient refuses oral potassium from this point onward. The patient was given another dose resulting in more gastric distress.

ETHICS WORKSHEET 2 ANSWERS

MATCH THE WORD TO THE DEFINITION

1. Credentialling:
2. Certification:
3. Licensure:
4. Autonomy:
5. Supervision:.
6. Beneficence:
7. Justice:
8. Nonmaleficence:
9. Unlicensed:
10. Delegation
11. Competence

   a. Self-determination and decision making
   b. Legal authority to perform medical interventions and procedures
   c. Actions for the welfare of others
   d. Fairness to all
   e. Qualification entitling the right to defined power
   f. Assignment of a task or mission
   g. Attesting to a level of achievement
   h. Lacking legal authority
   i. Do no harm
   j. Facilitates control
   k. Ability to perform efficiently

Answers:

1. __E____   2. _G_____   3. __B____   4. __A_____   5. __F_____
6. ___C_____ 7. __D_____   8. ___I___   9. ___H____   10. __J_____
11. __K_____

ETHICS WORKSHEET 3 answers

1. Research a bioethics topic, such as stem cells. List the ethical pros and cons of your chosen topic. Explain which side you favor and why.

2. Define autonomy: Ability to make independent actions

3. Explain how autonomy relates to nursing: Nurses assess the patient and make decisions based on those findings. For example. The nurse may chose to take an axillary temperature in the patient who has oral canker sores. This is a judgement made by the nurse.

4. Explain how autonomy relates to patient choices. The patient may refuse blood if their religion does not allow their members to accept blood transfusions. This is an independent action by the patient.

5. Define disclosure: Making information known. Giving the patient all available information so the patient can make an informed decision.

6. Explain the legal position of a nurse regarding informed consent for a patient who may become a research candidate: The patient must be informed of all potential risks and possibilities. The patient must made aware they may quit the research program at any time.

7. Define nonmaleficence: To do no harm.

8. Explain how non-maleficence plays a role in research or post operative care: Research is the attempt to prove a theory which may be to improve patient care. In this process, the doctors attempt to do no harm. Regarding the post-operative patient, the physician may deem not to order chemotherapy if the outcome would cause more discomfort and pain for a terminal condition. Thus, the doctor will do no harm.

9. Give an example of a situation in which a nurse may advocate for the patient: The nurse must represent the patient and the patient's wishes regarding care, visitors, and the patient's choices if the patient choses to refuse care. The family may not agree. The nurse will support the patient's choices.

10. List the people that maybe involved in making clinical decisions for a patient. Explain how they maybe come involved in the decision-making process: A legal power of attorney (POA) has a legal document explaining the limitation of the POA given by the patient. A guardian, if the guardian is the parents are legally able to make decisions for their child. A spouse may make decision for the married partner. A living will directs what clinical decisions may be made for the patient. An advanced directive also has guidance on clinical decisions.

11. Explain the self-determination act when the patient is mentally incompetent: Patient's with intellectual disabilities have the same right to self-determination as anyone else. However; if the disability is such that the mentally incompetent patient is unable to make appropriate decisions or understand the situation, a parent, guardian, POA, or court appointed POA may intervene.

12. Define integrity: being honest, having strong principals.

13. How does integrity affect the nurse when assuming the role of patient advocate? The nurse must follow the patient's desire and not make choices based on his/her personal principals. The patient trusts the nurse to be honest.

14. Is caring a legal or professional requirement for a nurse? Explain your answer. No, it is not a legal or professional requirement. However; without empathy or the ability to care for another the nursing intervention may not be as affective. Caring assists to build a trusting relationship between the nurse and the patient.

ETHICS WORKSHEET 4 answers

1. Define precedence: Taking priority.

2. How does precedence play a role in nursing? Give an example. . if staffing is short and the manager wants the nurses to take an additional patient for the shift, it would set precedence. Which means once it has been done once, it can be done again. The additional burden has taken priority over the paying someone overtime.

3. Define competence: The ability to perform a skill or task efficiently.

4. How does healthcare ensure the nurse is competent? Give an example. The facility may test the staff annually to ensure they can perform the skill or task efficiently.

5. Define assault: To verbalize the intent to commit an action that results in a threat to the patient

6. Define battery: Carrying through with a verbalized intent or the intentional act of causing physical harm to the patient.

7. Give an example of assault: Threatening to tie the patient in restraints if he doesn't stay in bed.

8. Give an example of battery: Tying the patient in restraints.

9. Give an example of false imprisonment of a patient: Tying the patient in restraints unnecessarily.

10. What is defamation? Stating false statements that may cause harm to a person's reputation.

11. Define HIPAA: The health insurance portability and accountability act which is a federal law the protects patient health information from disclosure with the patient's consent.

12. List five examples of how a nursing student can maintain HIPAA when participating in nursing clinical classes. Do not talk about the patient in public places. Use only initials when gathering information and writing it down. Do not take pictures of patient information. Do not tell others about your patient. Place any information that may breach HIPAA into the shredder prior to leaving the clinical class.

13. Define negligence: Failure to provide appropriate care and safety that another prudent nurse would have provided under the same situation.

14. Give an example of neglect: Failure to provide the patient with food or water.

15. Explain the relationship between neglect and malpractice: Although they may seem the same they are slightly different. Neglect is when harm is caused accidently. Malpractice is when harm occurs by a decision that the health care professional made and was aware the action could cause harm.

16. A patient's condition is terminal but the family wants everything done. To continue medical care would cause prolonged pain for the patient. Who should make the determination of ceasing further life-prolonging care if the patient is unable? The patient, if the patient is able to make their own decision. However; the doctor can decide continued intervention is futile and would only cause a painful death and therefore; could cease to order those interventions.

ETHICS WORKSHEET 5 answers

1. Using one of the included ethical dilemmas, explain what YOU would do ethically as a nurse for the patient.

    e. A suicidal patient
    f. A patient refusing a blood transfusion but will die without this intervention
    g. A 13-year-old wanting an abortion
    h. A patient seeking an assisted death

2. What is a living will? A written document stating the patient's medical interventions in the event the patient is unable to express their wishes.

3. What is medical power of attorney? Do they have limitations? Explain your answer: A medical power of attorney when a chosen person can make medical decisions for a patient when that patient is unable to make decisions. Yes, they have limitations. They can only make decisions on behalf of the patient's health. Medical power of attorney does not allow decisions to be made outside the scope of the document for health care proxy.

4. Choose one of the included scenarios. Explain how you would advocate for the patient if you were the assigned nurse.
    e. A patient that no longer wants her life prolonged by chemotherapy
    f. A patient with a living will that states no life support has severe pneumonia
    g. A patient with malignant gallstones who doesn't want surgery
    h. A ventilated brain-dead patient who is listed as an organ donor but the family refuses

5. List members of the healthcare team and a brief description of their role:
Charge nurse, accountability for assignments and ensuring the unit functions efficiently. The staff nurse, take care of assigned patients. Patient care technician, assists the nurse in the care of the patient. The doctor, assesses the patient and prescribes appropriate medical interventions. Respiratory therapist, assists to provide respiratory treatments or supplemental oxygen. Case worker, reviews the patient's chart to determine potential needs status post discharge. Pharmacist, ensures all medications are correctly available and compatible. Dietician, ensure the appropriate diet for the patient. Laboratory technician, provides phlebotomy services that adhere to correct patient to specimen collection. Reports laboratory results. Clergy, offers spiritual support (optional). Radiology technician, may need to take images of the patient. House keeper, keeps the hospital environment clean. Supply clerk, stocks the patient's needs. Security officers, ensure a safe environment.

6. Define collaboration: Participation that builds a good team.

7. How does collaboration with other healthcare team members play a role in the nurse-patient relationship? The healthcare team will communicate to ensure the appropriate healthcare member will offer input to ensure the best care and outcome for the patient.

8. A married couple choses to have the wife's eggs frozen. Years later, they are divorced. The wife wants the eggs destroyed. The husband wants the eggs to survive. Explain who decides reproductive rights and privileges. How does this play a role in ethical and legal issues. Research your state law on the matter.

9. The doctor writes an order. YOU as the nurse believes it is in error. Explain what, if anything, you can do: Contact the doctor and explain how you believe the order was an error. If the doctor believes it is correct and you, the nurse believes it is still in error, contact your charge nurse.

10. You are assigned a patient that states, "I only use osteopathic medications and methods." Explain what osteopathic is and it will affect your care of the patient. Osteopathic treats the whole patient and not "just the symptoms". They tend to use preventive interventions and treat the body as a whole. They have four units: the body, the person, the mind, and the spirit.

EYE 1 answers

1. List two types of macular degeneration. Give a brief description of each.

Dry and wet. Dry: the macula breaks down slowly resulting in loss of vision. Wet: Blood vessels grow abnormally beneath the retina. The blood leaks (wet) causing a blind spot in the visual field.

2. What are cataracts? A cataract occurs when the eyes lens becomes cloudy.

3. Listed below are three types of cataracts. List where each type forms.

Subcapsular	On the posterior side of the lens
Nuclear	At the nucleus of the lens
Cortical	Outside of the lens to the center

4. List risk factors for cataracts.

Diabetic patients
Patients that use steroids
Smoking
Excessive sunlight
obesity

5. Your patient has a visual opacity of the left eye. What do you assess the opacity to be?

It could be a posterior vitreous detachment (PVD), an infection, or eye injury.

6. List two risk factors for dry macular degeneration.

Smoking, hypertension, diet high in fats, and over the age of 50 years.

7. The doctor has performed cataract surgery on your patient. How would you prevent the patient from rubbing the surgical eye? By placing an eye shield over the post-operative eye.

EYE 2 answers

1. Briefly explain what may be diagnosed in the patient with increased intraocular pressure. Glaucoma is diagnosed when intraocular pressure increases in the eye. This pressure can damage the optic nerve.
2. What can cause increased intraocular pressure? Resistance or inability of the drainage canals to drain aqueous humor fluid.

3. List two types of glaucoma and give a brief definition of each.

a. Open-angle glaucoma	Aqueous humor is unable to drain via the eye's drainage canals. Pressure builds up in the eye. Slow onset
b. Closed-angle glaucoma	Sudden onset. The eyes dilate too quickly blocking the drainage canals resulting in pressure build up

4. What is a complication of untreated glaucoma? Vision loss or blindness. Both irreversible.

5. What is a Snellen chart? How is it used? A scale to measure visual acuity from a distance. The patients attempts to read the smallest letter to determine their clarity from a distance.

6. Define what each letter in PERRLA means.

P	pupils
E	equal
R	round
R	Reactive
L	To light
A	accommodation

FETUS 1 answers

1. What is an alpha fetoprotein test? Include what abnormal levels indicate in your response. The alpha fetoprotein test is a test performed during pregnancy that can determine the risk of birth defects in the baby. Normal levels for a neonate are 41,687 Ig/L. In a preterm infant the normal levels are 158,125 Ig/L.

2. What is an amniocentesis and when would it be considered? Amniocentesis is a test performed between 16 – 20 weeks gestation to determine fetal abnormalities. (Down syndrome, spina bifida, or cystic fibrosis).

3. What is the purpose of monitoring HCG (human chorionic gonadotrophin)? Monitoring HCG can assist to diagnose molar pregnancies, potential miscarriages, or other abnormal pregnancies.

4. What is the purpose of karyotyping? To assess if the infant has a full set of chromosomes.

5. List the risk of CVS (chorionic villus sampling). Bleeding, infection, or pregnancy loss.

6. When would an amniotic fluid aspiration be performed? At birth

7. List what may compromise a vaginal delivery. Cervix does not dilate, infant is in the wrong position, uterine rupture, umbilical cord prolapse, severe bleeding, or maternal hypertension

8. Explain what are Braxton Hicks contractions? False labor pains. Also called prodromal

9. How does the nurse know the fetus is progressing for delivery? The cervix is fully dilated. The cervix has effaced, and the fetus is in position.

10. What does it mean if the effacement is partial? The cervix has thinned but is only half way to becoming fully effaced.

11. At what stage of labor would an epidural be offered? When the cervix is dilated 4 – 6 centimeters.

12. What is an episiotomy and at what stage of labor may a mother require one? An episiotomy is a surgical cut made in the perineum to allow the vaginal opening to be wider for an easier birth.

13. At what stage of labor is the placenta expelled? The third stage

14. What is the purpose of a uterine massage? To prevent postpartum hemorrhage and stimulates the uterine to contract.

15. What is the purpose of the APGAR score? It is a test to see how will the baby tolerated the birthing process.

16. What is one of the biggest problem with a new born? aspiration

17. List interventions to prevent hypothermia of the infant. Clean with warm water. Cover the head. Wrap in warm blanket. Place in warm incubator.

18. When and why would the nurse need to monitor the infant's glucose levels? When the baby is two hours old and before feedings. Glucose is monitored for the first several days to ensure the baby is not hypoglycemic.

FLUIDS AND ELECTROLYTES 1 answers

1. Explain how fluids and electrolytes are distributed though out the body. Fluids move throughout the body because of osmotic pressure, hydrostatic pressure and osmosis. Electrolytes are moved the same way.

2. List three ways a patient may lose fluids. Vomiting, diarrhea, excessive sweating, or failure to take in fluids.

3. List two causes of electrolyte and fluid imbalance that may occur because of therapeutic treatment. The use of diuretics can cause the lose of fluids and electrolytes. A patient with a nasogastric tube to suction will lose fluids and electrolytes.

4. List the four main electrolytes in the body. Potassium, calcium, sodium, chloride, magnesium and bicarbonate.

5. What is the relationship between electrolytes and IV nutritional therapy? IV therapy is capable of delivering not only fluids and electrolytes but also nutrients directly into the blood stream.

6. Define the following.

topic	definition
osmosis	The movement of a solvent through a semipermeable membrane
diffusion	The movement of molecules from an area of higher concentration to an area of lower concentration
Active transport	Is when molecules may cross a cell membrane by use of energy
filtration	The removal of waste products through the kidneys

7. Explain the difference between sensible and insensible losses. Sensible losses are through the process of urination or defecation. Insensible losses are fluid losses through the act of sweating or respirations.

8. Explain how the kidney plays a role in the regulation of fluid and electrolytes. The kidneys can balance fluids and electrolytes through the filtering process.

9. Explain how hormones play a role in the regulation of fluid and electrolytes. The body produces the antidiuretic hormone which will signal the kidneys to reabsorb water and electrolytes during the urination process.

10. Explain the difference between isotonic, hypertonic, and hypotonic. Isotonic is the same solution as that of the body. Hypertonic means the fluid has a higher osmotic pressure than that of the body. Hypotonic means the fluid has a lower osmotic pressure than that of the body.

11. List the risks factors involved in fluid volume deficit. (remember injuries can play a part). Older adults may take a diuretic, have a progressive neurological disease (dementia), Children have a high metabolic rate and may not meet the needed requirements. Baby also have a high metabolic rate and are dependent on others for fluids.

12. List the risks factors involved in fluid volume excess.

    Hypernatremia, Head injury, heart disease, or hypervolemia.

FLUID AND ELECTROLYTES 2 answers

List the risk factors of the following electrolyte abnormalities.

1. Hyponatremia: ingesting too much water, or syndrome of inappropriate antidiuretic hormone.

2. Hypernatremia: elderly, diuretic therapy, neurological disorder (dementia),

3. Hypokalemia: diabetic ketoacidosis, diarrhea, or non-potassium sparing diuretic.

4. Hyperkalemia: renal failure. Consuming a diet rich in potassium.

5. Hypocalcemia: hypoparathyroidism or inadequate vitamin D.

6. Hypercalcemia: cancer or over active thyroid

7. Hypomagnesemia: alcoholism, malnutrition, or diabetes

8. Hypermagnesemia: chronic renal disease or hypothyroidism

9. Hypophosphatemia: vomiting, diarrhea, or alcoholism

10. Hyperphosphatemia: diabetes or obesity

List two risk factors or causes for each of the following conditions

1. Metabolic acidosis: aspirin over-dose or kidney failure

2. Metabolic alkalosis: Excessive use of antacids or decreased kidney perfusion

3. Respiratory acidosis: sleep apnea, drug overdose (suppressed respirations), COPD.

4. Respiratory alkalosis: Fever, pain, or hyperventilation

FLUID AND ELECTROLYTES 3 answers

1. List two ways to assess a patients hydration status. Skin tenting, dry mucous membranes, or weak thready pulse

2. Explain how fluid and electrolytes help to maintain the body's stable environment. The body's fluids and electrolytes move in and out of cells to maintain homeostasis.

3. List two diseases that may affect fluid and electrolyte balances. Anorexia, and burns

4. Give an example of a treatment in which the nurse must anticipate a potential fluid and electrolyte imbalance. Explain why this imbalance occurs. Administering a diuretic. The diuretic is given to remove fluid from the body via the urinary system. Often sodium or potassium are removed when the body eliminates the fluid.

5. Name two fluid compartments of the body and which electrolyte is of higher concentration. Intracellular (potassium) and extracellular (sodium).

6. List two areas of the body that contain extracellular fluid. The brain and spinal cord

7. List three locations in the body with transcellular fluid. Gastrointestinal tract, urinary bladder and the aqueous humor of the eye.

List the locations of the following. Draw an arrow to the correct answer	LOCATION
Interstitial fluid	Around the cells
Intravascular fluid	Within veins and arteries
Lymph fluid	Within the lymphatic vessels
transcellular	Aqueous humor of the eye

List if the following electrolytes are positive or negatively charged.	NEGATIVE OR POSITIVELY CHARGED
SODIUM	positive
POTASSIUM	Positive
CALCIUM	positive
MAGNESIUM	positive
CHLORIDE	negative

FOUNDATIONS IN NURSING WORKSHEET 1 answers

1. Define professionalism. Explain how to become a professional. Competent and skilled. Become educated

2. Define an occupation. What is the difference between an occupation and a profession? An occupation is on the job training of a specific task. A profession requires higher education

3. What is the definition of nursing per the American Nursing Association.

4. What is meant be the art of nursing? An art and science

5. What is meant by the science of nursing? Nursing involves learning and understanding the basic sciences and then applying that learning to their practices.

6. What type of nursing degree can a student attain from a community college? Associate of science degree.

7. What type of nursing degree can a student attain from a university? A bachelor of science in nursing

8. What is accreditation and how does it play a role in healthcare? Accreditation is a process that is determined by the state board of nursing to ensure the educational programs offered by the university or college meet the standard requirements. If accreditation is not met, it can alter funding.

9. Why is accreditation important when applying for a nursing program? If the university or college is not accredited, the school cannot secure federal funding, the reputation is lost, and the school may close.

10. What characteristics should a nurse possess? Explain your answer. Critical thinking, ability to communicate, time management, compassion, empathy, and honesty.

11. What is the purpose of nursing organizations? Advocates for nurses. Promotes higher standards for the nursing profession.

12. Who makes up the regulatory licensing boards? Representatives from leading organizations

13. List the various roles a nurse may choose to work. Bedside nurse, charge nurse, nurse manager, researcher, operating room nurse, emergency room nurse, flight nurse, cruise nurse, community health nurse, home health care nurse, nurse educator, diabetic educator, wound care nurse, nurse practitioner, nurse anesthetist, or midwife.

14. List the various types of healthcare services available in your community. (the student must answer this question based on their own community)

15. What is the nursing scope of practice? List the six factors in the scope of nursing. The actions that the nurses license permits that RN to perform. Assessment, diagnose, outcomes, planning, implementation and evaluation.

16. Explain what the duties of a nurse means and how it differs from obligation. Duties are the tasks the nurse has been trained to perform. Obligation is the legality to perform and complete those tasks.

17. What is the nursing process? A systematic guide for the nurse

18. List the steps of the nursing process. Assessment, diagnose, outcomes, planning, implementation and evaluation

19. What is the standards of nursing practice. Who, what, where, when, why and how.

FOUNDATIONS OF NURSING WORKSHEET 2 answers

1. How should a nurse introduce himself/herself to the patient? Greet the patient. Inform the patient of your name. Explain your role.

2. List several ways in which a nursing student or new nurse can promote or maintain patient dignity. Close the door. Pull the curtain. Keep the patient covered as much as possible. Ask the patient what name they wish to be called.

3. If the patient states, "I don't want a student nurse assigned to me," what should the student do? Let the patient know, you understand and will let your professor know. Notify your instructor.

4. Define holistic. Give an example of how a holistic problem may impact patient care. The whole patient is taken into account. The patient may be worried about finances. This may impact decisions on health care chosen by the patient.

5. How is competence determined in a health care professional? Annual competency testing

6. What are professional boundaries? Give an example. The legal framework that demonstrates professional limitations. A bedside nurse may not be able to work in a critical care area due to limited certification.

7. What is therapeutic communication? Explain why it is important in nursing. The ability to communicate with the patient using verbal or non-verbal methods. It is important for the nurse to assess and gather data adequately.

8. List four different types of therapeutic communication techniques. Give an example of each.

    Silence: sitting nearby quietly but offering unspoken support.
    Active listening: Listening to the patient and showing active participation by nodding the head or providing input when appropriate.
    Restating: Repeating what the patient said back to him to confirm.
    Reflection: Encouraging the patient to determine their own solution

9. Explain the relationship between nursing and honesty. Patient must trust the nurse. The nurse must demonstrate honesty in order for the patient to build trust.

10. How does truth play a role in healthcare? The patient must know the truth in order to make an informed consent

11. Define culture. A way of life for a specific population

12. How does culture play a role in healthcare? The patient may have cultural beliefs that need to be considered when caring for the patient in order to make adequate health care choices.

13. Can social media play a role in healthcare? Explain your answer Yes. Social media can assist to make the public aware of potential health news.

14. Define discrimination. Unjust treatment

15. List two examples of discrimination in healthcare. Race, color, age, or sex

16. Explain how professional behavior in nursing plays a role in how nurses are viewed by the public.

    If a nurse does not act professional, it reflects on the entire nursing profession.

FOUNDATIONS OF NURSING WORKSHEET 3 answers

1. What is a nurse? A person who assists to prevent diseases and promote healthy recovery when the patient presents with an illness or injury.

2. How can a nurse use warm and caring communication techniques to improve patient participation in their care? Give an example. By using touch. A hand on a hand. A hand on a shoulder.

3. How can non-verbal communication cause an issue in patient participation? Explain your answer. If the nurse demonstrates non-verbal communication that may indicate to the patient that they are not important, it can cause disharmony in the patient to nurse relationship. An example, is the nurse looking at her watch and edging toward the door while the patient is speaking.

4. Explain why the patient is given a patient-bill-of-rights on admission. To notify the patient of their rights to have access to information so they can make an informed decision.

5. Explain the difference between rights and responsibilities. Rights are legal freedoms. Responsibilities are actions or tasks we should do.

6. How does the patient-bill-of-rights empower the patient and his/her family? The bill of rights gives the patient or the patient's family the right to communicate with health care providers.

7. What is a nursing plan of care? A documented framework that determines the patient's needs and a planned collaboration between the patient's health care team to promote a progressive action plan to promote health or improvement in health.

8. Explain the importance of the nursing plan of care. Include how collaboration plays a role. The nursing care plan records the patient's needs and progress. It keeps the patient's health care team informed of the needs and progress of the patient's health.

9. Is it true, once a nurse completes the nursing program and passes the state board of nursing examination, there is no further educational requirements needed? Explain your answer. No. There are always changes in health care. Research allows improvement in care. It is the nurses responsibility to keep up-to-date of new interventions. Continuing education is often mandatory in each state in order to renew the nursing licensure.

10. Is it true, when an ethical issue arises, the nurse can take time to contemplate the situation before determining an intervention? Explain your response. The nurse must follow protocols to report any ethical situation. Often ethics dilemmas have life and death decisions and ethical situations should be addressed in a timely manner.

11. List ways in which to facilitate discussions when an ethical and clinical conflict occurs. Assess the situation and determine everyone who may play a role in the ethical dilemma. Set a time to have a meeting with all parties. In the hospital, the ethics committee may need to participate in the meeting. Use active listening. Attempt to come up with an agreeable plan.

12. List ways to teach a new nurse how to become a patient advocate. Give an example of each response.

    a. Promote patient safety (the first priority). Bed locked in low position
    b. Allow the patient his/her patient rights. To make choices in their plan of care
    c. Educate the patient on the pros and cons of treatment choices

13. List examples of non-therapeutic communication phrases that can block effective communication between the nurse and the patient.
    a. The nurse giving his/her opinion instead of allowing the patient to make their own decision
    b. Coercion of the patient to do what the nurse "thinks" is best
    c. The nurse demonstrating judgmental behaviors

14. Explain why healthcare systems are focusing on patient safety. Give an example of a way in which the healthcare system promotes a safe environment. The goal of health care is to "do no harm". Health care attempts to prevent injuries and adverse events. Using "time out", or ensuring safety measures are in place assist to promote safety. Having the call bell in reach. The bed in low and locked position.

15. Give an example of how a nurse can avoid non-therapeutic communication. A nurse may brush off a patient's concern. "You have nothing to worry about, the doctor is a good doctor." This does not allow the patient's concerns to be addressed.

FOUNDATIONS OF NURSING WORKSHEET 4 answers

1. Your patient asks you, "what is my diagnosis?" Can you, as the assigned nurse give your patient their diagnosis, prognosis, and potential treatment plan? Explain your answer. The doctor is responsible for notifying the patient of their diagnose, prognosis and treatment plan. However; the nurse often is asked to participate in the discussions due their presence in the care of the patient.

2. Often patients and their families feel vulnerable and powerless. Their lack of knowledge of the healthcare arena, routines, and protocols makes them fearful. Why must the nurse interpret the patient and family's position and ensure other healthcare team members recognize the needs and preferences of the patient and family? The nurse must act in the role of patient advocate to ensure the patient's desires are represented.

3. Explain why the nurse must maintain professional boundaries. Professional boundaries provide the nurse with a better position in which to provide care that benefits the patient's needs.

4. List issues of cultural diversity that may arise in healthcare. Stereotyping, language barriers, race, ethnicity, socioeconomic status, sexual orientation, gender identity, or disabilities.

5. How can the nurse or healthcare system ensure cultural diversity is incorporated into the patient's plan of care? Give an example. By learning more about different cultures. Often middle eastern female patients cannot have a male nurse.

6. Explain how you, as the nurse, can facilitate coordination of the interdisciplinary team. Provide input and feedback during daily rounds. Document in a timely manner to ensure the interdisciplinary team members have current patient data to make decisions.

7. As a patient's health improves, it is often necessary to transfer the patient to an external healthcare facility. Explain how the interdisciplinary team must work together to ensure this process. The doctor must document the patient's progress and needs. The case worker must work with the patient and the patient's family for a facility that they agree is appropriate. The pharmacist must have all current medications and dosages up-to-date in the patient's record. The assigned nurse must report to the nurse at the accepting facility.

8. Explain the difference between managed care, a health maintenance organization (HMO) and a preferred provider organization (PPO). Managed care is quality health care provided a contained cost. A health maintenance organization is an insurance that limits care to those in their network. A medical plan that is chosen by the patient that will allow care provided by those in their chosen network.

9. Explain what the federal false claims act is and how it pertains to kick backs, false claims in billing, and self-referrals. The federal false claims act allows the government to file claims against those who attempt to defraud by billing for goods or services never provided. A kickback is when someone attains a benefit by participating in a bribery like agreement.

10. What is risk management? Often a process that identifies and monitors situations that may pose a risk resulting in financial liability.

11. What is the relationship between risk management and nursing? The nurse may assess a risk in his/her practice which would need to be addressed to risk management. Such as a fall or a medication error.

12. What is the difference between people skills and technical skills? People skills is the ability to communicate and basically get along with others. Technical skills are skills necessary to do the assigned job.

13. What is quality improvement or quality assurance and how does it play a role in patient care? Quality improvement is the act of incorporating evidence-based research into the practice of health care to improve the care to the patient. Quality assurance is the action of meeting the standards of care.

FOUNDATIONS OF NURSING WORKSHEET 5 answers

1. What is evidence-based-practice (EBP)? EBP is providing quality care based on knowledge obtained from research.

2. Where did the nursing profession originally get its skills and knowledge? Originally the care was learned from nuns and monks. Later as nursing progressed, the profession obtained many of its skills and knowledge from the medical profession

3. Why is EBP important in nursing? Because keeping current of EBP, it promotes better outcome for the patients.

4. List the interdisciplinary team and their role in patient rounds.
    a. Assigned nurse: provides brief pass medical history and current issues that need to be addressed.
    b. The charge nurse: Must be kept abreast of the patients status
    c. The physician: Determines if current medical regime is appropriate or needs changes
    d. The respiratory therapist: Available in the event supplemental oxygen, treatments, or respiratory monitoring is required.
    e. Pharmacist: ensures cost effective medications (generic) and ensures all prescribed medications are compatible
    f. Case manager: Assists in planning discharge in the event home health or rehabilitation facility may be needed.
    g. Dietician: Ensures adequate dietary calories are planned and consumed.

5. What is informatics? Digital technology that provides healthcare the availability to document via computer. Patient's electronic medical records.

6. Has informatics improved healthcare? Explain your response. Yes. A digital medical record can be accessed by multiple interdisciplinary team members at the same time. It can be accessed from remote destinations.

7. List two new challenges informatics bring to HIPAA regulations. Ensuring any record sent to a remote area is received at the intended site. Computer breaches. Computers left open with someone not authorized to view the patient record.

8. Explain the relationship between quality improvement and EBP. Evidence-based practices when incorporating new justified improvements can assist to provide better quality patient outcomes.

9. How can the care based on EBP be documented in the patient's plan of care as a positive performance outcome? Documenting in the patients nursing care plan any provided care can be reviewed and determined if the care provided assisted in a positive outcome.

10. Problem-solving is a skill the nurse must learn. A problem may occur due to poor communication, culture, or patient beliefs. Give an example of situation that may occur based on the three issues listed and how you as the nurse would problem solve the situation.
    a. Using closed-ended questions reducing the information the nurse receives. Clarify the information to ensure all the data is understood.
    b. Culture: failure to learn more about the patient's culture may prevent the nurse from understanding the view of the patient. Ask the patient more about their culture and how they anticipate their culture playing a role in their care.
    c. The patient may have religious beliefs that do not correlate with the plan of care. Ensure the nurse understands the patient's beliefs and advocates for those beliefs.

G.I. SYSTEM 1 answers

1. Your patient has been diagnosed with a G.I. Bleed. The stool is black, and tarry. Based on your findings, is this an upper G.I. bleed or a lower G.I. Bleed? Explain your rationale.

> Upper G.I. Bleed as the blood has gone through the digestive process resulting in black stools

2. What information would you want to gather from the GI bleed patient?

Information	Rationale
a. When did it start b. What medications are you taking C. How much blood have you expelled	a. Timely diagnosis is important to determine severity b. Some medications may cause bleeding c. Knowing the amount can also assist to determine the severity of the situation

3. List five interventions that would be appropriate for a patient with an upper G.I. bleed.

Interventions	Rationale
a. Obtaining a CBC b. Monitor vital signs frequently c. Inserting a nasogastric tube d. Sending a specimen for occult blood e. Initiate an NPO status f. Maintain bedrest	a. Determine hemoglobin level b. Vitals signs can alert the nurse to hypovolemic shock c. An NGT can assist to lavage and monitor the bleed d. An occult blood specimen can confirm a GIB e. An NPO status is necessary to prevent dislodgement of a clot in the event the GIB is healing f. Bedrest can promote safety in the event of low blood pressure or a syncopal episode.

G.I. SYSTEM 2 answers

1. A patient admitted status post (S/P) motor vehicle crash (MVC). The patient's car was T-boned. From the force, the patient's car then spun and hit a light pole. The patient is complaining of left upper quad pain. Lists the possible causes of this patient's pain.

A splenic injury. Broken ribs. Muscular pain.

2. What tests might be appropriate for this patient? Include your rationale for each test.

Test	rationale
A computed tomography (CT)	A CT scan can detect organ injuries, determine hematomas or blood in the abdomen

3. What past medical history might you want to include in the patient's medical record?

Information	Rationale
a. Health issues that may contribute to the MVC b. Current medications c. If the patient had a history of substance abuse	a. Some health issues may cause driving issues, such as seizures, hyperglycemia, narcolepsy, or hypertension b. Some medications may cause drowsiness c. If the patient drinks alcohol in excess or takes non-prescribed drugs it can result in drowsiness or lack of judgement.

GI SYSTEM 3 answers

1. Your patient with a nasogastric tube is complaining of nausea. What interventions will you provide?

Interventions	Rationale
a. Check patency of the nasogastric tube b. Ensure the NGT is in the appropriate place c. Ensure the suction is working appropriately d. Administer an antiemetic	a. A blocked NGT will not allow GI contents from being removed b. An NGT that has migrated, may not be able to suction appropriately c. Suction that is not working properly can not remove the gastric secretions allowing build up and nausea d. Giving an antiemetic may assist the patient to feel less nauseated.

2. The patient fell off a high ladder and is diagnosed with a spinal injury. The doctor orders the patient to be logrolled. What is logrolled and why is it ordered?

The patient is logrolled which means to keep the spine aligned while repositioning the patient. This procedure will prevent injuries to the spine.

3. The doctor orders your patient to be in the supine position. The patient begins to complain that the medication has made him nauseated. What interventions will you provide? Explain your rationale.

Intervention	Rationale
Tilt the entire bed (head up and foot down.	This will maintain the patient in the supine position while bringing the head upward to prevent aspiration
Administer an antiemetic	This will assist to relieve the nausea
Notify the doctor	If previous interventions do not relieve the problem, notify the doctor

4. The pulse oximetry alarm on the contracted patient with a continuous tube feeding is sounding. You enter the room and see the patient's mouth is full of tube feeding. List your actions based on priority.

> Stop the tube feeding. Turn the patient onto their side. Suction their mouth. Notify the doctor of the situation. If the tube feeding is via an NGT, assess placement of the NGT tube and residual if in the proper place. If via a PEG, assess residual.

Gastrointestinal 4 answers

Match the following.

GI subject	Definition
1. Colectomy (F)	a. blocked colon
2. total colectomy (G)	b. inflammation of the bowel resulting in sores
3. partial colectomy (H)	c. inflammation of the bowels
4. hemicolectomy (D)	d. removal of the left or right colon
5. proctocolectomy (E)	e. entire colon and rectum removed
6. bowel obstruction (A)	f. Surgical removal of the colon or a section removed
7. Crohn's disease (C)	g. Entire colon removed
8. Ulcerative colitis (B)	h. part of colon removed

1. What is a P.E.G.? A percutaneous gastrostomy tube used for feeding

2. 7. What is a nasogastric tube (NGT) and why is it ordered? Nasogastric tube placed into the stomach to remove the contents of the stomach. It may be to decompress, assess for GIB, or to prevent distention status post GI surgery.

3. Can a patient receive medications and tube feeding via a nasogastric tube? Yes

4. How is nasogastric tube placement initially confirmed? With a 10 ml air bolus and auscultation

5. Why is an X-ray required to confirm the placement of a nasogastric tube? To ensure placement.

6. A patient with an NGT is coughing a lot. What would be the nurse's concern? That the NGT dislodged.

7. The patient who has been receiving a continuous tube feeding via a NGT has a distended abdomen. What would you assess? Residual tube feeding amount. Hold if greater than 250 mL.

HEALTH AND WELLNESS answers

1. List at minimal six aspects of health and wellness.

    a. Physical health
    b. Financial health
    c. Emotional health
    d. Spiritual health
    e. Occupational health
    f. Social health

2. List two ways a patient's health can be affected.

    a. Physical environment
    b. stress

3. List three of each of the following factors that affect health.

Modifiable	Non-modifiable
Quit smoking	Age
Healthy diet	Gender
Exercise	race

4. List ways in which a patient may meet a desired outcome. Participate in the plan of care. Adhere to the prescribed diet. Exercise. Eliminate stress.

5. Explain what is the illness to wellness continuum. _The relationship that reflects preventative intervention in the promotion of health and its effectiveness

6. Define illness.
   A period of unwellness

7. List obstacles that may prevent a patient from complying with necessary health changes or lifestyle changes.
    a. Lack of understanding
    b. Lack of financial ability
    c. Lack of transportation

HORMONE 1 answers

1. List the signs and symptoms of Cushing's syndrome and Cushing's disease. List the differences as well as similar signs and symptoms.

Health issue	Signs/symptoms	Similar signs	Different signs/causes
Cushing's syndrome	High cortisol levels Hypertension Diabetes II Weight gain Fatigue Purple striae	Slow wound healing Fatty lump on upper back Easy bruising Moon face	Exogenous steroids
Cushing's disease	High cortisol levels Hypertension Diabetes II Weight gain Fatigue Purple striae	Slow wound healing Fatty lump on upper back Easy bruising Moon face	Endogenous steriods

2. The patient says he is between jobs and can't afford the steroid medication. He has one week's worth of medication remaining. He asks you if he can just stop or does he need to keep taking the steroid medication. How would you respond? Explain your rationale.

Steroids must be tapered off in order to allow time for the adrenal glands to function adequately

3. List the differences between the two hormones below.

Hormone	Benefits	Side effects
Glucocorticoid	Assist to reduce inflammation	hyperglycemia
Mineralocorticoid	Assists to promote sodium reabsorption in the kidneys	hypertension

INFANT 1 answers

1. When assessing the pulse of the newborn infant, list the sites and expected heart rate. The pulse of an infant is taken at the brachial artery. The heart rate is 70 – 190 beats per minute.

2. Would you expect to hear infant bowel sounds immediately after birth? Explain your response. Bowel sounds are not present at birth but are usually auscultated after 15 minutes status post birth.

3. What is the purpose of eye prophylaxis? To prevent eye infections that may occur through a sexually transmitted disease, such as gonorrhea or chlamydia.

4. What is the purpose of phytonadione? It is given to assist with the blood clotting factors.

5. What may cause jaundice in an infant? Excessive bilirubin in the blood.

6. What are Mongolian spots? Congenital birthmarks of infants with Asian or African parents

7. What are typical assessment factors in an infant examination? At birth, the Apgar score. Typical assessment factors include weight and head circumference, fontanelles, and vital signs.

8. What are the characteristics of fetal alcohol syndrome? Facial anomalies, physical deformities, mental retardation.

9. When should the infant have their first stool? Within the first 24 hours or before day two.

10. What are the characteristics of an infant born to a substance addicted mother? The baby may present with withdrawal symptoms, be irritable or have feeding issues.

11. Briefly explain how a blood sample is obtained from an infant. Via heel punctures

12. What is the purpose of an incubator? Provides an environment that permits temperature, oxygen, and light adjustments to meet the infants needs.

13. Why are caps placed on the infant's head? Infants loose body heat through the head. The caps attempt to prevent this loss.

14. What considerations should be taken when bathing the infant? Be mindful that the infant doesn't get cold. Ensure to hold the infant to prevent harm

INFECTION WORKSHEET answers

Match the following:

			Match letter with number
i. Abscess	1. Cell death		a. 3
ii. Exudate	2. A vulnerability		b. 4
iii. Transudate	3. Accumulation of purulent material		c. 6
iv. Inflammation	4. Fluid that seeps from blood vessels or organs		d. 8
v. Necrosis	5. Intervention to reduce risk of transmission		e. 1
vi. Nosocomial	6. Fluids that pass through a membrane		f. 10
vii. Purulent	7. Discharge		g. 7
viii. Vector	8. A reaction to tissue	h.9	
ix. Susceptibility	9. Transmits a pathogen	i.2	
x. Standard precautions	10. hospital acquired	j.5	

Match the precaution			
i. airborne	1. MRSA, VRE, ESBL, C-diff, Conjunctivitis, RSV, impetigo, lice, and scabies	a. 2	
ii. Droplet	2. Chickenpox, measles, tuberculosis	b. 3	
iii. Contact	3. Whooping cough, pneumonia, diphtheria, adenovirus, meningococcal, mumps, and scarlet fever	c. 1	

INTEGUMENTARY SYSTEM 1 answers

1. Define Exudate: Fluid that leaks out of blood vessels due to the inflammatory process
2. Define transudate: Fluids that leak out of blood vessels due to a change in hydrostatic pressures
3. Explain the difference between a bedsore and a pressure ulcer.
   They are the same.

4. List the anticipated duration of healing in the following pressure-ulcers stages.

Stage 1	If discovered early, it will take a few days to heal
Stage 2	It can take a period of a few days to weeks to heal
Stage 3	It can take months to heal (approx.. 4 months)
Stage 4	It may take ½ a year to heal

5. Explain how a pressure ulcer is measured? First by the length of the wound (using a clock, from 12 to 6), then measure the width (from 9 to 3), then measure the depth by using a moistened sterile cotton-tipped applicator and measure it against a disposable sterile ruler gauge. A pre-marked probe may be available to use as well.

6. List what should be assessed each time a dressing is changed. Amount of drainage, color, odor, and type of drainage (serous, bloody, etc.). Color of the wound bed and cellular growth. Any necrosis or eschar.

7. What is eschar and how is it is treated? Eschar is dry, dead tissue. It is removed using an enzymatic ointment (prescribed) or surgically removed.

8. What color is granulation tissue? Healthy granulation tissue is pink in color

9. You are precepting. You must explain to the student nurse what tunneling means. Explain what tunneling means how is it measured? Tunneling is the wound which "tunnels" underneath the skin surface. It is measured using a moist sterile cotton-tipped applicator or a pre-marked probe.

INTEGUMENTARY SYSTEM 2 answers

1. Explain epidermis and why it's important. The epidermis the outer most layer of the skin that provides the body's first line of protection

2. Explain the health benefits of darker skin. Darker skin provides more protection from the sun's UV radiation.

3. What are Merkel cells? Merkel cells are cells which provide the body with the sensation of touch

4. What is the primary function of skin? The primary function of skin is protect the body from external threats.

5. Can skin be a delivery system for medication? Explain your response. Yes. Topical medications are absorbed.

6. Define endogenous and its relationship with vitamin D. Exogenous means originating from outside the body. Vitamin D is made by the body when UV radiation is absorbed through the skin.

7. List potential causes of the following skin colors.

Jaundice	Liver failure or gall stones
Delayed wound healing	Inappropriate vitamin A levels. Diabetes.
Cyanosis	Heart failure. Respiratory failure
Pallor	Anemia. Excessive blood loss

8. Define the following.
   Psoriasis: A skin disease characterized by scaly patches.
   Pruritis: Excessive itching of the skin.
   Ecchymosis: Bruising.

9. List what changes in the skin that should be assessed. If the skin is discolored, becomes excessively warm or cold, or if it becomes hard.

INTEGUMENTARY SYSTEM 3 answers

1. What is an angioma? A benign tumor

2. List what is petechiae and its cause. Petechiae is a rash caused by hemorrhaging into the skin. Excessive pressure, such as frequent vomiting.

3. What is the difference between turgor and texture of the skin? Turgor reflects the elasticity of the skin. Texture reflects the condition of the skin.

4. Your surgical patient has a history of keloids. What is a keloid? A keloid is scar tissue where the skin grows beyond the site of injury or surgery. The site presents as a abnormal growth above the injured site.

5. Your patient loves to lie in the sun. On cloudy days, the patient uses a tanning bed. Could this practice cause problems with the skin? Explain your answer. This behavior can increase the risk of developing skin cancer.

6. Some medications can potentiate the suns effects on the skin. Explain what this means and what, if anything, can be done. Photosensitivity is the term used. The sun may cause rashes, or cause a change in the skin.

7. What is contact dermatitis? An allergic reaction to something that has come in contact to the skin

8. Explain why the following are important when assessing a mole.

Asymmetry	A sign of a melanoma
Border irregularity	Melanomas have uneven borders
Color change	It is the first sign of a melanoma
Diameter of 6 mm or larger	Most melanomas are greater than 6 mm
Evolving	Evolving means change. The mole may grow, change colors, or even disappear

9. What is a melanoma? A type of skin cancer

10. What is the most common cause of skin cancer? Basal cell carcinoma.

LAW WORKSHEET 1 answers

1. Your patient's family member was pushing buttons on the patient's bed and inadvertently raised the height of the bed, while you were attending to another patient. The patient did not use the call bell, attempted to get up to go to the bathroom, and fell. After examination, the patient had a broken femur. The family has initiated a lawsuit for malpractice. Is this case malpractice? Explain your answer. No. Malpractice is injury that occurs when care is given. This situation was caused by the family.

2. What are the four factors that must be met to be considered malpractice. Professional duty to the patient, breach of duty, injury resulted because of breach of this duty, and injuries or damages that had incurred.

3. What is meant by "scope of practice" and what determines the scope? Explain your response. The scope of practice is the permitted activities determined by licensure, education, and training. The state board of nursing determines the scope of practice.

4. Define the standards of practice. Standards of practice are the policies and protocols that determine how the nurse may practice based on his/her education, training, and licensure.

5. What is the nurse practice act? The state law that determines the responsibilities and duties of a nurse.

6. Explain why a graduate student must pass the state board of nursing exam. To ensure the student meets the competency required.

7. Who is the nursing license meant to protect? Explain your rationale. The state board of nursing protects the public. It ensures those who receive the license is competent to practice.

8. The electrical cord on the bed has exposed wires. Occasionally, a spark can be seen. The patient care technician states, "Your patient complained he received a shock when his foot touched the bed frame and he thinks his life was put in danger. The patient is talking about suing." Who is responsible for the functionality of the equipment used? Explain your response. The nurse is responsible for all equipment used.

9. What is a tort? A act that results injury or harm to a person or their property

10. What is a deposition? A out-of-court testimony.

11. What is a defendant? A person accused of a wrong

12. What is a complainant? A person who makes a complaint resulting in a lawsuit.

13. Explain the process of a medical lawsuit from the initial filing to the result. A complaint files the complaint. If the defendant fights the complaint, a plead is made. Discovery occurs. A trial begins. The verdict. If not satisfied, either the complainant or the defendant may file an appeal.

14. Define litigation and how does it affect professional nursing. Litigation is the act of attempting to settle a dispute using the legal system.

15. What is a subpoena? A legal order that requires the person (whose is named in the subpoena) to appear in court

16. What is an affidavit? A written document that verifies truth to the content of the document by the person whose signature is on the document.

LAW WORKSHEET 2 answers

1. Define law. A system of rules which direct the actions of the population of society.

2. What is the main purpose of a law? The main purpose of the law is to establish and ensure the rights of a population

3. What, if any, would be the penalties for violating the law? Punishment, which may include a blemish on their record, paying a fine, serve jail time, or lose a privilege.

4. Define ethics. The right or wrong of situation.

5. What is the main purpose of ethics? Provide a framework to guide in making decisions

6. What, if any would be the penalties for violating ethics? Loss of job, loss of licensure, fines, or jail time.

7. What are moral values? The personal guidelines to assist when making a decision between right and wrong.

8. What is the main purpose of moral values? Assisting to make the right choice in a moral situation

9. What, if any, would be the penalties for violating moral values? Moral values are personal. Inputting ones own moral values into a healthcare situation may cause a conflict of interest, if those values go against the patient's choices. This can result in loss of job, loss of licensure, a fine, or jail time

10. Define protocol. Rules that guide conduct or procedures.

11. What is the main purpose of protocols? Protocols serve as a consistent guide

12. What, if any, would be the penalties for violating protocols? It would depend on the protocol. For example, sharing patient information is a breach of HIPAA and can result in loss of job and a fine.

13. How are the laws enforced by the state board of nursing? The state board can take disciplinary actions by suspending a nursing license or completely loosing the nursing licensure.

14. Compare the difference between morals and ethics. Ethics is determined by the healthcare system and must be followed. Morals is the persons own personal choice in a given situation.

15. Define Values. A person's personal standards

16. How do morals and values relate to ethics in nursing? Morals and values are the personal preferences of a nurse, however; ethics is a specific action guided by rules of healthcare .

17. How do religious beliefs play a role in ethics? Religious beliefs may influence and guide a person, whereas, ethics is guided by rules of healthcare.

18. During the Covid-19 pandemic medical supplies were not readily available. A shortage of ventilators was of concern. Who shall be given the use of a ventilator knowing the person not chosen would or could die? Explain your answer.

MAKE-UP ASSIGNMENTS answers

1. Explain what evidence-based-practice is and how it pertains to bedside nursing. Evidence-based practice is researched theories that prove best outcomes. These outcomes incorporated into bedside nursing practice has proven to improve patient outcomes.
2. What is diversity in nursing and how does it play a key role? Diversity is actively including people of different ethnical backgrounds into the group. Diversity ensures the best care for all people. Diversity strengthens the practice of nursing by encouraging people of different ethnical backgrounds from education other nurses.
3. Must laboratory results be known prior to medication administration? Does pharmacy play a role in this interaction? Explain your response. Yes, If a medication may affect a change in the patient's laboratory results. For example, if the patient has a low potassium level and a diuretic is given. The diuretic may cause the patient's potassium level to become too low causing a lethal cardiac rhythm. The pharmacist must monitor the patient for some laboratory levels when dispensing medications. Such as patients who are polypharmacy. Multiple medications may cause renal issues.
4. List three types of nurses that are currently in the nursing profession. Include their unique characteristics in your response. Licensed practical nurse (LPN): Hard-working nurses who usually work in SNL facilities.
Registered nurse (RN): Work at bedside. May become certified in their area of practice.
RN-NP: registered nurse practitioner. Provides care similar to a physician under the licensure of a doctor.
5. List the various nursing positions or nursing jobs. Include how education plays a role in these various positions. **(the student should research this)**

6. Should nurses get involved in legislation? Include in your response how the state board of nursing plays a role. Yes. Nurses should have a voice. By becoming actively involved in legislation, the state board of nursing can extend the scope of practice of nurses in the blossoming fields of nursing. Nurses can also lead in nursing organizations that fight for nursing rights.
7. Explain how euthanasia differs from comfort care. Euthanasia is assisting a patient to die based on their wish to no longer live. Comfort care is providing comfort to the dying patient while they are actively in the dying process.
8. Does the academic arena of nursing differ from bedside nursing in relationship to salaries? Explain your response. Yes. Academic nurses (nurse faculty) are often paid less than bedside nurses. This seems odd since it takes a higher education to become a nursing instructor.

9. It has been stated that, "nursing eats their young." What is the meaning of this statement. Do you believe it is true? Explain your response. This statement refers to nurse bullying. Today's healthcare environment attempts to promote a healthy collaborative environment.

10. Should continuing educational units be a mandatory requirement for the nursing profession? Explain your response. Yes. New knowledge and skills arise consistently. The nurse should incorporate best practices and knowledge into his/her practice.

MAKE-UP ASSIGNMENT 2 answers

(no answers available for this assignment as it is student driven)

Research one nursing article (peer-reviewed) that pertains to your chosen field of nursing. Write a summary of the article. Include why this field is your chosen field and how this article supports your choice

MAKE-UP ASSIGNMENT 3 answers

(there are no answers for this assignment as it is student driven)

Make up an examine question for each of the following health disparities.

1. Cerebral vascular accident
2. Closed head injury
3. Myocardial infarction
4. Angina
5. Pneumonia
6. Gastrointestinal bleed
7. Small bowel obstruction
8. Renal failure
9. Pressure ulcers
10. Fractured hip

Match the following work sheet answers

Review Maslow's hierarchy. Match the following

		Match column 2 with column 1
A. Physiological	a. family	a. C
	b. acceptance	b. E
	c. sleep	c. A
B. Safety and security	d. intimacy	d. C
	e. food	e. A
	f. achievement	f. D
	g. confidence	g. D
C. Love and belonging	h. health	h. B
	i. breathing	i. A
	j. morality	j. E
D. Self-esteem	k. shelter	k. A
	l. friendship	l. C
	m. water	m. A
E. Self-actualization	n. job	n. B
	o. clothing	o. A

MATERNITY 1 answers

Match the following.
1. Creamy appearing breast milk
2. Breast milk that ceases approximately three weeks after the birth of the new born
3. Breast milk that contains 90% water
4. Breast milk that provides immunity for newborn
5. Breast milk that contains lactose and has high levels of fat

Match with definition above and place your answer in the appropriate space below

   A. Colostrum   B. Transitional   C. Mature

1.__A____   2.____B____   3. ___C____   4. ___A_____   5. _____C___

- ❖ Explain the psychological difference between breast milk and formula in mother- baby bonding. Mothers that breast feed share touch and eye contact with the infant. This process often is associated with a closer mother-baby bonding. Bottle feeding, especially when the child is older, does not have that close touch connection.

- ❖ Explain what is meant when the milk is letting down. It is a response that results in the causing the breast milk to begin flowing.

- ❖ Briefly explain how a new mother can determine her baby is obtaining milk when placed to the breast. There may be milk on the side of the babies mouth. The baby can be seen swallowing. The breast becomes less firm. The baby has 5 or more wet diapers daily. The baby is gaining weight.

MATERNITY 2 answers

1. Briefly compare and contrast cultural breast feeding practices for the following:

    d. Hispanic: Blend both breast feeding and bottle feeding
    e. Asian: breast feed. Feel comfortable breast feeding in public
    f. African American: Breast feed to build a strong bond between mother and infant

2. List two reasons breast milk production may cease. Low milk supply. Irregular or infrequent feedings. Some medications may cause breast milk production to cease.

3. Can breast milk be refrigerated? If yes, how many days may breast milk be refrigerated and still be considered usable? Yes. Up to a maximum of four days

4. Can breast milk be frozen? Explain your response. Yes. Breast milk may be frozen up to a maximum of 12 months

5. Can the consumption of breast milk cause a change in the color of the baby's stool? Breast milk may change to a light tan or yellow color. Hints of green have also been noted.

6. Explain the relationship between breast feeding and wet diapers. Include why this relationship is important. If an infant is breast feeding adequately and consuming enough milk, it will result in more wet diapers. The baby should also show weight gain

7. A mother must take medication for a sinus infection. Will drugs be present in the breast milk? Explain your response. Yes, decongestants pass into the breast milk. Mothers are educated not to breast feed within two hours of taking a decongestant.

8. Can consumed food cause a change in the color of breast milk? Explain your response. Yes. Foods with artificial dyes, or foods with high carotene content can change the color of breast milk.

9. Can food and beverages that the mother consumes cause the baby to NOT want to nurse? Explain your response. Yes. Caffeine can make its way into the breast milk. Some additional foods and beverages may cause the baby not want to nurse. Garlic, peppermint, and chocolate.

MATERNITY 3 answers

1. Briefly describe the stages of labor. Stage I Cervix is dilated and effacement . Stage II: expulsion of the fetus. Stage III: placental delivery. Stage IV: Recovery

2. Briefly describe the phases of labor. Phase I: the latent phase. Contractions begin and the cervix begins to dilate. Phase II: The active phase. The contractions are regular and the cervix has dilated greater than 5 centimeters. . Phase III: This is the phase of intense labor. Contractions are back-to-back and last for a longer duration.

3. Briefly describe the differences between true labor and false labor. True labor is determined with regular contractions that get closer together, stronger and will not cease with rest. False labor or Braxton Hicks contractions are irregular. Their duration may be irregular or regular but cease with position changes or rest.

4. Are there signs that precede labor? Explain your response. Yes. Nesting: a surge in energy. Lightening: feeling like the baby dropped into birthing position.

5. Define: latent, active, and transition. Latent: dormant . Active: ready to engage. Transition: changing from one condition to another.

6. What is the difference between internal and external fetal monitoring? External monitoring is a method of monitoring the fetus. This method could be affected by movement from the mother or fetus. External monitoring can be used after four months of pregnancy. Internal monitoring

can only be used when active labor is occurring and the amniotic sac has ruptured. Internal monitoring provides a more accurate monitoring of the fetal heart rate.

7. Give an example when internal fetal monitoring may be required. When the fetal heart rate demonstrates distress.

8. Give an example when external fetal monitoring may be required. To monitor the fetal heart rate during labor.

9. What is the importance of baseline changes in fetal monitoring? Accelerations or decelerations of the fetal heart rate can indicate fetal distress, such as bradycardia or hypoxia.

10. Define: Accelerations as it pertains to fetal monitoring. Accelerations in the heart rate are normal during labor.

11. Briefly explain the difference between early, variable, and late deceleration in fetal monitoring. Early deceleration may represent uterine contractions during active labor. Variable: May represent disrupted blood flow through the umbilical cord (cord compression). Late deceleration: May represent fetal acidemia due to cord compression. This is an emergency.

12. Explain the difference between voluntary and involuntary uterine contractions. Voluntary is when the mother "pushes". Involuntary is the uterus contracting in reaction to the natural birthing process.

13. What is uterine fatigue? Include an example of what may cause uterine fatigue. Uterine fatigue, also known as uterine atony, is when the uterine is weak after child birth and the muscles do not contract resulting in bleeding. This can be caused by prolonged labor or the use of oxytocin.

14. Explain how the mother's position may affect the strength and frequency of contractions. A mother in the supine position will feel more pain, have a tendency for hypotension, and slower delivery. When the mother walks, stands, or sits, these positions assist with contractions.

15. Briefly explain the relationship between hydration and uterine activity. Dehydration may cause Braxton Hick contractions. It may also cause low amniotic fluid levels.

16. List three factors that may influence the pushing efforts of the mother. Fatigue, pain, and anxiety.

MATERNITY 4 answers

1. Define the following:

    j. Fontanels: Soft spot at the junction of bone in the infants skull

    k. Breech: Buttocks or legs emerge first during birth

    l. Transverse: The fetus is a horizonal position in the uterus instead of vertical

    m. Attitude: This refers to fetal position

    n. Position: The position of the fetus in relationship to the mother during labor

    o. Contraction pattern: This is defining the contractions. They may be regular or irregular. The duration is also considered.

    p. Effacement: When the cervix thins and prepares for childbirth

    q. Cervical dilation: The opening of the cervix in preparation for child birth.

    r. Cephalic: Refers to the head

2. Name the sutures of the fetus: Coronal, sagittal, lambdoid, and frontal.

3. Briefly explain the relationship between the position of fetus and level of pain experienced by the mother. As the birthing process continues, the contractions become more intense (painful) and the duration may be longer.

4. List ways in which the nurse can determine the birth is eminent. Loss of the mucus plug, amniotic sac breaks, contractions begin, or crowning of the skull.

5. List ways in which the nurse may held make the mother more comfortable during labor. Encourage the mother to rest between contractions. To get in a comfortable position. Empty her bladder frequently. Offer ice chips.

MATERNITY 5 answers

1. Match the following:

To be defined	definition	Correct response
a. Presumptive signs of pregnancy	1. Lack of menses	a. __2__
b. Probable signs of pregnancy	2. Signs experienced by the woman herself	b. __6__
c. Positive signs of pregnancy	3. Softening of the cervix	c. __4__
d. Amenorrhea	4. Signs apparent on physical exam by the doctor	d. __1__
e. Goodell's sign	5. Bluish vaginal tissue	e. __3__
f. Chadwick's sign	6. Signs that determine a positive pregnancy	f. __5__

2. What is supine hypotension syndrome and what intervention must the nurse provide when the woman presents with supine hypotension syndrome? This is inferior vena cava compression syndrome. Hypotension occurs when the mother is in a supine position and the uterus compresses the inferior vena cava. The nurse must turn the mother onto her side.

3. In the table below, list one change that occurs in the pregnant woman

Breast	Breast become tender and enlarge
Blood volume	The body produces more blood to meet the needed demands of mother and baby
Respiratory	The body's demand for oxygen increases with pregnancy.

Gastrointestinal	The abdomen enlarges. The mother may become nauseated. Become constipated. Have gastric reflux.
Cardiac	Pregnancy makes the heart work harder. There is an increase in blood volume requiring the heart rate to increase.
urinary	Frequent urination

MATERNITY 6 answers

Match the word	To the definition	Correct answer
1. Apgar score	a. Vaginal discharge status post (S/P) delivery consisting of mucous, blood and tissue	1. E
2. hyperbilirubinemia	B. Flexion of the legs and arms of the infant when startled by loud noise(s)	2. D
3. Lochia	C. Incision to avoid tearing or laceration of the perineum	3. A
4. Acrocyanosis	d. Elevated levels of insufficient conjugated serum bilirubin	4. G
5. Moro's reflex	e. Scale on which the condition of the newborn is assessed immediately after birth	5. B
6. Areola	f. Breakdown product of hemoglobin that produces an orange pigment	6. H
7. Episiotomy	g. Bluish color of infants hands and feet at the time of birth to 10 days after time of birth	7. C
8. Bilirubin	h. Darker tissue surrounding the nipple	8. F

MATERNITY 7 answers

POSTPARTUM

1. Briefly explain why the new mother experiences "afterpains" postpartum. They are normal pains the mother may experience for several days postpartum due to the uterus returning to pre-pregnancy size.

2. Explain the changes in the lochia from rubra, serosa, and alba. Include why quarter size clots should be reported in your response. Lochia rubra is deep red three days post-partum then begins to lighten (lochia serosa) post-partum days 4 to 10. The lochia then changes to a light brown or creamy white ten days to up to six weeks post-partum. Quarter size or larger clots must be reported to the doctor. This may indicate hemorrhage.

3. Why should the breasts be assessed for redness, heat, pain, and engorgement? These are signs of mastitis (an infection).

4. Why is it important to assess the level of the fundus? To ensure the uterus is gradually decreasing.

5. What is the purpose of assessing the amount and type of lochia? To ensure there is no infection or hemorrhage.

6. Your patient who has had an epidural removed complains of a headache. Is a headache normal after the removal of an epidural? Explain your response. No. A head ache is not normal and may be a sign of a spinal headache.

7. You are assessing the fundus and notice it is off-center. What can cause this to occur? If the bladder is full, the fundus may be moved off-center.

8. Your patient states she heard an old wife's tale that a woman doesn't ovulate when breast feeding and therefore, cannot get pregnant. Is this true? Explain your response. It is true that ovulation does not occur during breast feeding if certain criteria are met.

9. Explain why the doctor maybe concerned that the mother is Rh negative and her baby is Rh positive. The mother's immune system will see the Rh positive fetal cells as an invader and destroy the fetal blood cells.

10. Briefly explain which hormone influences milk let down and what action stimulates the hormone. Oxytocin stimulates the let-down of milk during breast feeding. Prolactin triggers milk production.

MATERNITY 8 answers

1. What is meant by maternal-infant attachment? The bonding between mother and infant

2. Explain what occurs during the taking-in phase. The new mother needs rest and depends on others to meet her needs.

3. Explain what occurs during the taking-hold phase. The new mother begins to adapt to her new role. She demonstrates independent and dependent roles.

4. Explain what occurs during the letting-go phase. The new mother adapts to parenthood and assumes full responsibility.

5. Your patient returns to for her postpartum check-up. She admits that she noticed significant hair loss. Briefly explain what may cause this to occur. Estrogen and progesterone decline postpartum which can trigger hair loss.

6. List four ways to resolve hard and tender engorged breast. Encourage frequent emptying of the breast. Warm compresses can be applied. Pump the breast or manually expel the breast milk.

7. List ways to help prevent engorgement in the non-breastfeeding mother. Encourage the mother to wear a tight, supportive bra. Apply ice packs. Avoid stimulation of the breast.

8. Explain the relationship of lactogenesis and the hormones: estrogen, progesterone, prolactin, and oxytocin. Lactogenesis is the onset of breast milk. During this process, estrogen and progesterone levels decline. Prolactin triggers the milk production and oxytocin triggers the letting-down of the milk.

9. List a minimal of four benefits to breastfeeding. (Include both maternal and infant benefits in your response). For the mother, it prevents ovulation, may trigger weight loss, may prevent cancer of the breast and uterus. For the infant, breast feeding stimulates a bonding between mother and infant. Provides optimal nutrition and offers immunity.

10. What is the concern if the patient is diagnosed with uterine atony? Hemorrhaging.

11. List why your patient may experience hypotension. Uterine hemorrhaging.

12. Briefly explain why there is an increased risk of thromboembolism in your postpartum patient. Do to the hypercoagulable state, the mother may experience blood clots. Also from decreased mobility, clots may form.

13. List two reasons breast feeding is contraindicated. If the mother has HIV or the infant is extremely ill.

14. What is the purpose of a lactation consultant? To assist the mother during the transition from breast to bottle. The lactation consultant can assist the mother to help reduce her milk supply.

MATERNITY 9 answers

1. List five causes that may inhibit involution status post-delivery. Dystocia, hypocalcemia, metritis, endometritis, blood clots, and infection.

2. What duration would you expect to see lochia rubra? Immediately postpartum for 3 days.

3. What duration would you expect to see lochia serosa? 3 to days postpartum

4. What duration would you expect to see lochia alba? 10 days to 6 weeks postpartum

5. There is an offensive odor to the lochia. What may be the cause? An infection

6. What types of analgesia may be used during labor? Include how the analgesia may affect the mother or the infant in your response. Opioids may be used but may suppress the respiratory system of the mother and infant. Opioids may also slow the labor process. An epidural may be used with an opioid.

7. Briefly define what is a support person and their role during the labor process. A support person to assist the mother during her birthing process. Their role is offer emotional support. Assist to keep the mother comfortable.

8. Can the absence of a support person affect the mother who is in labor? Explain your response. Yes. Lack of a support person has been linked to post-partum depression.

9. How can the fetal heart rate be obtained during labor? Using an external fetal monitor

10. How long do contractions continue after the birth of the baby? Contractions continue for up to 10 days postpartum to ensure the uterus returns its pre-pregnancy size.

11. Define multipara. A woman who has had two or more pregnancies with viable births

12. Define Para. Para is defined as number of births.

13. What concerns may present in the laboring substance abuse mother? The mother may not tolerate the pain. The fetus may be developmentally disabled. The fetus may have substance withdrawal.

14. List two reasons a caesarian birth may be required. When there are multiple fetus and a vaginal delivery may place the fetuses or mother at risk. If there is a problem with the umbilical cord or placenta. The position of the fetus may compromise the fetus or mother's safety.

15. What is Lamaze? Is a method of techniques that teach physical and psychological ways to prepare for child birth.

16. What is Naegele's rule? A way to calculate the date of delivery

17. Why is it important to complete a cultural assessment? Because the mother's culture may affect what the mother will expect during her pregnancy, child birth, and rearing the child.

18. Explain the relationship between late deceleration and fetal distress. Late decelerations that are recorded on a fetal monitor may indict the fetus is in distress and may require a caesarean section delivery.

MEDICATION 1 answers

(answers are student specific and therefore cannot be provided here)

1. List three medication your patient has been prescribed or have your instructor assign three medications. Complete the following for each medication.

Medication name	Classification of each medication listed

Medication name	Indications for each medication

Medication name	Usual dosage of each medication

Medication name	Side effects or adverse reaction of each

2. Your patient has been prescribed a short and long-acting insulin. Complete the following.

Name a short-acting insulin	Name a long-acting insulin

List the onset of the short-acting insulin	List the onset of the long-acting insulin

List the peak time of the short-acting insulin	List the peak time of the long-acting insulin

List one insulin the short-acting insulin can be mixed with and one it cannot be mixed with	List one insulin the long-acting insulin can be mixed with and one it cannot be mixed with

MENTAL HEALTH 1 answers

Match the following

Word	Match the correct Definition	
1. Repression	A. c	d. returning to less developed state
2. Suppression	B. e	e. separating from conscious awareness
3. Projection	C. f	c. inhibiting feelings
4. Regression	D. a	d. justifying
5. Rationalization	E. d	e. act of stopping self
6. Disassociation	F. b	f. attributes given to another
7. Reaction formation	G. g	g. express opposite of true feelings

	A. grandiose	1. b	a. Believing self is dead
	B. Delusions	2. d	b. Believing self is important
	C. Nihilistic	3. a	c. believes others are against
	D. Persecution	4. c	d. False beliefs

MENTAL HEALTH 2 answers

Match the following suicidal risk to the correct definition

Level	Correct level	definition
1. high risk	A. c	a. The patient has a plan, less likely to elope, past suicidal plans, monitor frequently
2. moderate risk	B. a	b. No plan. Zero, one or two symptoms.
3. low risk	B. b	c. Patient has a lethal plan. Denies any hope

Fill in the blank from the options from the table below.

1. Desires to be treated as the opposite sex from which the patient has been given at birth.
   _____D_____.

2. Disturbed thoughts and auditory hallucinations that may be a risk for violence to self or others.
   _____C_____.

3. May have increased libido, elation, fragmented thoughts, flight of ideas, and change in sleep and appetite. ____A_____.

4. Failure to pay attention. Avoids tasks that are considered disliked. Fails to listen.
   _____B_____.

A.	Bipolar
B.	Attention deficit disorder
C.	Schizophrenic
D.	Gender dysphoria

MUSCULOSKELETAL 1 answers

Define the following and explain its importance in a skeletal injury:

    a. Pain: physical state of discomfort. Injury to a bone may cause acute pain.

    b. Pulse: palpable method of assessing the heart rate. The lack of a pulse is an emergent situation and may result in amputation

    c. Paresthesia: the sensation of tingling that does not occur from an external stimulus. Paresthesia is a sign of pressure on a nerve

    d. Paralysis: loss of movement. An injury can result in paralysis of the muscles, or spine.

    e. Pallor: Pale in color. Reduced blood flow from an injury can be caused by the injury to a blood vessel, or swelling which impedes circulation

2. List two acute orthopedic emergencies. Explain why they are emergencies.

    a. Open fracture. This is an emergency as it exposes the body to infection, may impede circulation.

    b. Compression syndrome: Compression syndrome is injury to an extremity that causes swelling and the skin works as a tourniquet, impeding blood flow.

3. Match the fracture to its definition

Fracture	Definition
1. Open fracture/compound	a. Fracture of bone but bone does not move or misalign
2. Greenstick fracture	b. Fracture that runs horizonal to bone
3. Transverse fracture	c. Fracture resulting with bone breaking through skin.
4. Spiral fracture	d. Fracture of bone but fracture does not extend through bone
5. Non-displaced fracture	e. A twisting motion of bone with fracture

1.___C_____ 2. ___D____ 3. ____B_____ 4. __E_____ 5. ____A_____

4.. List three most common reasons for fractures.

a. A fall
b. Motor vehicle crash
c. Abuse

5. What are shin splints? Can shin splints develop into fractures? Explain your answer. Shin splints occur when repetitive stress is placed on the shin bones which result in pain. If not allowed to heal, the shin splints can result in stress fractures.

MUSCULOSKELETAL 2 answers

1. Why is there a concern for compartment syndrome when there is a limb injury? The injury may result in swelling. The swelling can impede blood flow jeopardizing the injured limb.

2. When the patient has been diagnosed with compartment syndrome, what intervention should be implemented? Notify the doctor immediately. A fasciotomy must be done.

3. The patient with a compartment syndrome says the doctor instructed him to keep his leg at the level of his heart? The wants to know why. Briefly explain what your answer to this patient would be. Elevating the limb would decrease blood flow. Allowing the limb to be lower than the heart could increase the pressure.

4. What is buck's traction? A form of traction that aligns and immobilizes the injured limb.

5. What type of injury would buck's traction be used for? For hip fractures, or femur and pelvic fractures.

6. What is the difference between an open and a closed fracture? An open fracture is when the bone protrudes through the skin. A closed fracture is when the bone is broken by the skin remains intact.

7. What is an immobilizer? A removable device used to support and maintain immobility.

8. What is pin care and how often should it be performed? The cleansing of the metal pins of a fixator to prevent infection.

9. When should a back brace be applied? With the patient sitting or lying? The patient should be lying when the brace is applied.

10. Briefly explain how a sling should be positioned for the patient with a broken clavicle. The affected arm should be placed in the sling, then the shoulder strap should be placed in the appropriate position and secured.

11. What is the risk of immobility when the patient is on strict bedrest. Muscle atrophy, pressure ulcers, and blood clots.

12. List two benefits of increased mobility for the hospitalized patient. Preventing health issues such as atrophy, pressure ulcers, and blood clots, and earlier discharge.

13. What is deconditioning and how does hospitalization play a role in its potential occurrence as well as its prevention. Deconditioning is the process in which physical changes occur from immobility. Muscle atrophy can occur. Hospitals that place the patient on complete bed rest, and do not provide active or passive range of motion contribute to the deconditioning

14. Briefly explain the relationship between immobility and respiratory complications. Immobility does not allow adequate ventilation which may result in pneumonia.

MUSCULOSKELETAL 3 answers

Match the following topic with the correct definition

Topic	definition
1. Scoliosis	a. Genu valgum
2. Kyphosis	b. Dorsal flexion that may be temporary or permanent
3. Foot drop	c. Over curvature of the thoracic vertebra
4. Knock knees	d. Lateral curvature of the spine

1. __d__ 2. _c_ 3. __b__ 4. __a__

2. What is an abductor pillow? A support that is secured between the patient's legs to stabilize the body.

3. What condition post operatively would you use an abductor pillow? A fractured hip

4. What could be done if a "baby" toe is broken? Tape the baby toe to the toe next to you.

5. What is meant by cast care? Keeping the cast clean and dry.

6. Why would it be important for the nurse to assess the pulse and/or skin of the extremity with a cast? To ensure there is no swelling causing perfusion problems

7. Can a patient with a cast take a bath or shower? Explain your response. No. The cast could become moist which can compromise the integrity of the cast.

8. Should the patient with a broken clavicle, sleep with their sling in place? Yes, for support.

9. What is a halo brace? A brace that secures the head and neck in a fixed position to allow healing.

10. What is a cervical brace and when would it be used? A brace that supports the neck. It is used to prevent movement of the neck to allow healing of an injury.

11. What is whiplash? Injury of the neck that often occurs from rapid movement of the neck from forward to backward motion.

12. What is traction and when would it be used. Traction is a device used to align the body by pulling on the body part. Buck's traction is one type of traction.

NEUROLOGY 1 answers

1. List what neurological functions may be assessed in a neurological assessment.

Mental status exam (LOC)	Sensory exam
PERRLA	Reflexes exam
Bilateral grip strength	Cranial nerves exam
Motor exam (ROM)	Gait (if able)

2. List procedures that may be used to determine an ischemic stroke or cerebral aneurysm.
   Non-contrast computed tomography (CT) of the head, MRI, Lumbar puncture, or cerebral angiogram.

3. List the purpose of an E.E.G. (electroencephalography). Give two health issues that an E.E.G. may be used to diagnose.
   Seizures, epilepsy, brain tumors, and can be used for sleep disorders.

4. What is intracranial pressure (ICP) monitoring and what are the normal values.
   ICP normal values are 7 – 15 mm Hg (in supine position)
   CPP normal values are 60 – 100 mm Hg
   Remember MAP – ICP = CPP

5. What is the true name of a "spinal tap" and what is its purpose?
   A lumbar puncture. A lumbar puncture is used to diagnose meningitis

6. When would a "spinal tap" be contraindicated? Explain your answer. A spinal tap would be contraindicated if the patient had increased intracranial pressure or injury to the spine. A lumbar puncture would reduce the amount of cerebral spinal fluid which in turn can cause the brain to herniate and potentially result in death.

NEUROLOGY 2 answers

1. What is meningitis? Meningitis is inflammation of the meninges that surround the brain and the spinal cord
2. List at minimum two types of meningitis.
   Viral and bacterial meningitis
3. List two objective signs that when tested are positive in meningitis.

a.	fever
b.	vomiting

4. What procedure can be performed to confirm meningitis?
   A lumbar puncture
5. List a potential complication of meningitis.
   Loss of hearing, seizures, generalized weakness, impaired vision and speech.
6. What is a seizure?
   A seizure is erratic electrical activity of brain cells that result in abnormal muscular movements.
7. Define epilepsy.
   A disorder of the brain that presents with seizures.
8. List causes for a seizure.

a.. hyperthermia	b. meningitis
c. Head injury that injures the brain	d. hypernatremia
e. encephalitis	f. epilepsy

NEUROLOGY 3 answers

1. Give a brief description of each type of seizure listed below.

SEIZURE	DESCRIPTION
General	Abnormal electrical activity of the neurons which results in a seizure affecting both hemispheres of the brain
Tonic	Sudden rigidity of the extremities or trunk of the body.
Clonic	Jerking motions of the extremities. May occur on one or both sides of the body
Myoclonic	Uncontrolled muscle movement on one or both sides of the body but there is no change in consciousness
Complex	Staring episode that may last for a duration of 30 seconds to 2 minutes.
Simple	Seizure only affects a select small area of the brain and does not influence awareness

2. List safety precautions for a seizure patient.

   g. Keep bed in low position and locked position
   h. Remove items that may cause harm (sharp corners of night stands)
   i. Rail pads
   j. Refrain from having hot foods or liquids near the patient
   k. Shower instead of taking a bath
   l. Ensure doctor approves ability to drive

3. What patient teaching would you give a seizure patient regarding the following?

ISSUE	TEACHING
Drinking alcohol with antiseizure medication	Alcohol may potentiate the seizure medication and cause excessive drowsiness
Driving and frequent seizure activities	The MVA may prohibit someone who has frequent seizures from driving
Antiseizure medication and oral care	Antiseizure medications can cause inflammation of the gums resulting in bleeding gums or gum disease
Water and fire safety	Never swim alone or without a life guard. It is suggested to wear a flotation device while swimming

NEUROLOGICAL 4 answers

1. List a symptom of each of the following stages of Parkinson's disease.

STAGE 1	Tremors on one side of the body. There may be changes in posture, walking & facial expressions
STAGE 2	Rigidity. Tremors worsen
STAGE 3	Unsteady when standing. Falling may occur
STAGE 4	Requires equipment to assist to stand or walk. Requires help with ADL
STAGE 5	Increased stiffness. Becomes bedridden or wheel chair bound. Requires around the clock care.

2. List five physical findings that a nurse would observe in a Parkinson's disease patient.

    f. tremors
    g. Forward posture
    h. Shuffling gait
    i. Rigidity
    j. Drooling
    k. Frozen facial expressions

3. Is Alzheimer's disease reversible? Explain your response. NO. Alzheimer's disease is not reversible. There are changes in the brain which include amyloid plaques and tau tangles. Neurons dies and the brain begins to shrink.

4. List an example of each of the stages of Alzheimer's disease.

Stage 1: normal function	Symptoms have not appeared
Stage 2: very mild	Slight forgetfulness
Stage 3: mild	Definite memory problems.
Stage 4: Moderate	Memory loss worsens. Confusion noted
Stage 5: Moderate severe	Needs assistance. No longer independent. May have delusions or hallucinations
Stage 6: Severe	Symptoms become more severe. May not be able to communicate needs
Stage 7: Late-Stage	Lack of ability to stand or walk. May be on bedrest.

5. List safety interventions for the Alzheimer's disease patient.
    f. Ensure the door is locked and cannot be opened by the patient
    g. Ensure interior doors cannot be locked. The patient may lock themselves inside a room or closet.
    h. Cover electrical outlets. It is suggested to use childproof plugs
    i. Provide appropriate lighting
    j. Avoid using throw rugs.
    k. Use night lights in hallways and bathrooms
    l. Do not keep any hazardous materials, such as medications, bleach, etc. where the patient may have access.
    m. Evaluate patient appropriately to ensure safety measure apply. Such as preventing the confused patient from turning on the stove, turning on hot water, or

NEUROLOGY 5 answers

1. What is the disease described below? Multiple sclerosis
An autoimmune disease which demonstrates damaged myelinated sheaths in the central nervous system

2. What would bring this patient into the emergency room?
   Vision changes or balance issues bring the patient to the emergency room
3. What would be an anticipated medication for this disease? Solumedrol and immunosuppressive drug
4. What tests or procedures would you expect for this patient and why? An MRI can determine damage or scarring of the brain.
5. What health care team members would you anticipate would be on this patient's case? Neurologist, Rehabilitation doctor, nurse, patient care technician, clergy, pharmacist, and dietician.
6. What safety interventions should be implemented for this patient? At the patient's home, a ramp for a wheel chair and a keyless entry system for when the patient has generalized weakness. Easy to use handle grips for utensils. Keep items in easy reach. Avoid throw rugs or items that may cause falls. Hand rails on BOTH sides of the stairs or install a stair lift.
7. What patient teaching would be needed for this patient. Make certain to cover safety, medication, and mobility in your response. Patient education should include the progression of the disease and how it may affect activities of daily living. Safety should be a priority. Medications should be discussed with the patient. Steroids can raise blood sugar levels. Medication changes can affect the patients overall health status. Mobility will decrease as the disease progresses. Planning ahead will assist the patient to be able to be more self-independent for a longer period of time.
8. When would you anticipate the patient would be cleared for discharge to home or transferred to a skilled nursing inpatient facility (SNIF)? When the patient is able to care for self or have appropriate care for activities of daily living.

NEUROLOGY 6 answers

> 1. What is the disease described below? Amyotrophic lateral sclerosis (ALS) also known as Lou Gehrig's disease
>
> Disease of upper and lower motor neurons that progress to muscular atrophy, paralysis, then death

2. What would bring this patient into the emergency room?
   Dysphagia, dysarthria, or dyspnea
3. What would be an anticipated medication for this disease?
   Glutamate blockers that inhibit the neurotransmitter glutamate (Riluzole). Muscle relaxers to reduce muscle spasticity (Baclofen).
4. What tests or procedures would you expect for this patient and why?
   An electromyography (EMG) and nerve conduction study (NCS) to determine muscle and nerve functions.
5. What deficiency may resemble or cause neurological symptoms that can be mistaken for ALS?
   Vitamin B12 deficiency. A vitamin B12 deficit can result in muscle weakness.
6. What health care team members would you anticipate would be on this patient's case?
   Neurologist, physical therapist, respiratory therapist, dietitian, speech and occupational therapist, nurse, mental health therapist, and clergy.

7. What safety interventions should be implemented for this patient?
   Monitor for breathing or swallowing complications. Due to respiratory muscle weakness, the patient's ability to breath may become life-threatening. The patient's ability to swallow saliva may also become a risk for aspiration. As the patient's condition progressively deteriorates, assist with ADL. If the patient becomes totally dependent on a care provider, the patient may also need a ventilator to ensure adequate oxygenation. A tube may be placed for feeding. (NGT or PEG). Skin must be given adequate consideration as the patient is unable to move, pressure ulcers can develop.

8. What patient teaching would be needed for this patient. Make certain to cover safety, medication, and mobility in your response.
   When the diagnosis is made, the patient should be informed of the disease and it's progression. The patient should communicate their status honestly to ensure safety from falls, choking, the ability to speak, and personal care are addressed to ensure safety. The patient should be educated on the medications that are prescribed and why they are prescribed, the dosage, frequency, and time of day to be taken. The caregiver should also be informed of any and all information to ensure adequate monitoring and care.
9. When would you anticipate the patient would be cleared for discharge to home or transferred to a skilled nursing inpatient facility (SNIF)? Where the patient is discharged depends on the patient's level of progression, as well as personal preference. A patient may wish to hire healthcare workers to be available around the clock at their own home.

NEUROLOGY 7 answers

1. What is the disease described below? Myasthenia gravis
Autoimmune disease in which there is a loss of acetylcholine receptors at the neuromuscular junction

2. What would bring this patient into the emergency room?
   The patient may have trouble swallowing, visual problems, or muscle weakness.
3. What would be an anticipated medication for this disease?
   Pyridostigmine is given to promote electrical signals to the muscles and nerves. Mestinon which is a cholinesterase inhibitor. Corticosteroids such as prednisone are often prescribed to assist to block the immune system.
4. What tests or procedures would you expect for this patient and why? The doctor may draw blood to test for antibodies. A level of acetylcholine receptor antibodies in the blood specimen can help determine the myasthenia gravis diagnosis. A CT scan or MRI can be assess the thymus. As with ALS, an electromyography (EMG) test may be ordered to test the electrical activity of the muscles and nerves.
5. What health care team members would you anticipate would be on this patient's case?
   A neurologist, ophthalmologist, neuromuscular doctor, a dietician, physical therapy, speech and occupational therapist, mental health therapist, and nurse.
6. What safety interventions should be implemented for this patient?
   Monitor the patients airway. Muscle weakness may cause swallowing and aspiration issues. Educate the patient to do the more difficult task early while energy is at its best. Avoid heat. Hot climates can worsen symptoms.
7. What patient teaching would be needed for this patient. Make certain to cover safety, medication, and mobility in your response.
   A regular exercise regime can help keep the muscle strength and tone to prevent falls. Monitor for swallowing difficulties or cough. The duration of effectiveness of Pyridostigmine is short and multiple doses throughout the day will be needed. Myasthenia gravis has no cure but the presenting symptoms can be controlled with medication, exercise, and treatment.
8. What treatments may be included for myasthenia gravis?
   Plasmapheresis may be prescribed. Plasmapheresis is similar to dialysis as it removes abnormal antibodies from the blood. The patient will receive a blood transfusion to ensure normal antibodies for the transfused blood. IV infusion of immunoglobulin can also help by reducing the immune systems attack on the body's nervous system. A thymectomy, the surgical removal of the thymus gland may be done to remove any tumors that may present.
9. When would you anticipate the patient would be cleared for discharge to home or transferred to a skilled nursing inpatient facility (SNIF)?
   The patient would be discharged when the patient's has overcome the critical issue in which they were admitted. The patient may be discharged to a SNF if the patient requires additional therapy that may not be available at the patient's home.

NEUROLOGY 8 answers

1. What characteristics does multiple sclerosis (MS), Amyotrophic lateral sclerosis (ALS), and Myasthenia Gravis (MG) have in common?

    They all have muscle weaknesses. Monitoring of the airway is a priority. Risk for injury due to falls secondary from weakness can also be a common characteristic.

2. Explain the difference between relapsing and remission.

    During a relapse, the patient's symptoms become worse. During a remission the patient's symptoms improve partially or completely.

3. List a minimum of two risk factors that may trigger a relapse in multiple sclerosis.
   An infection and stress can trigger a relapse.

4. Which neurosensory disorder may present with Uhthoff's sign?
   Multiple sclerosis may temporarily worsen with Uhthoff's sign.

5. What is Uhthoff's sign? The worsening of the patient's neurological function due to increased core temperature.

6. Define the following:
    i. Dysarthria: Difficulty speaking. May be slow or slurred words.
    j. Dysphagia: difficulty swallowing.
    k. Expressive aphagia: the patient understands what is said but unable to clearly speak the response.
    l. Agnosia: Patient is unable to recognize or identify objects
    m. Spatial Neglect: Inability to sense, respond, or orient due to damage to the neural network.
    n. Receptive aphagia : Impaired ability to comprehend language.
    o. Hemiplegia: One side of the patient is paralyzed.
    p. Hemiparesis: One side of the patient's body is weak or inability of the patient to move one side of the body.

NEUROLOGY 9 answers

1. List two or more reasons a patient may complain of a headache.

    f. Constipation
    g. Stress
    h. Sinus allergies
    i. Dehydration
    j. Side-effect of medication

2. Define the difference between a migraine and a cluster headache.

Migraine	Cluster headache
A migraine is throbbing pain that occurs on one side of the head. Migraines build up slowly and have a long duration.	A cluster headache, comes on quickly with sharp pain. Usually the pain is behind the eye(s). The cluster headache may be intermittent.

3. List the symptoms the patient may complain to have occurred due to a headache.

Pain behind the eye. Throbbing pain on one side of the head. Sharp pain on one side of the Head. Photophobia.

4. Define the following stages of a headache.

Prodromal	The phase of the headache that occurs a day or two before the headache occurs. May include mood change and low energy.
Aura	Flashing lights or visual disturbances that occur before the headache occurs.
Second stage	This is the stage in which the aura occurs
Third stage	Photophobia, smells and sounds worsen the headache pain.
Recovery stage	Also known as the postdrome phase, the patient is fatigued and can last 1 to 2 days post headache.

5. List actions that may worsen a headache. Lights, sounds, and smells.

6. Are there foods that might trigger a migraine? If so, explain why and list the food. Yes. Caffeine, alcohol, Aged cheese and foods made with nitrates.

NEUROLOGY 10 answers

1. List the different classifications of head injury.

Diffuse axonal injury
Hemorrhage
Contusion
Concussion
Focal injury
edema

2. List two areas that may bleed from a head injury.

Epidural bleed
Subdural bleed

3. When a patient is admitted for a head injury, what other precautions should the nurse take?

Spinal precautions Seizure precautions Aspiration precautions

4. Explain what is meant by the golden hour when a patient is brought into the emergency room with a head injury.
The first sixty minutes after the head injury occurs. Healthcare must stop further damage (from bleeding or swelling), provide surgical intervention, or appropriate treatment to prevent worsening of the condition.
5. Why are the cranial nerves tested in a neurological assessment?
The cranial nerves are tested to assess for any worsening of the neurological state.
6. When you are assessing your febrile patient, you notice nuchal rigidity. What is nuchal rigidity and what does it indicate?

Nuchal rigidity is stiffness of the neck (when the neck is flexed). May be due to bacterial meningitis.

NEUROLOGY 11 answers

1. What may cause an increase in intracranial pressure?

A brain hemorrhage
A tumor
High blood pressure
Cerebral vascular accident
Aneurysm
Edema (from trauma)

2. List several interventions that the nurse may implement to reduce intracranial pressure.

Raise the head of the bed
Provide a quiet environment
Low light environment
Administer medication (pain medication, antihypertensive, mannitol, or Decadron)

3. What is the Monroe-Kellie Doctrine?

   Brain tissue, cerebral spinal fluid, and intracranial blood. The increase in one, usually results in the reduction of the remaining two.

4. Explain the process of brain herniation.

   Pressures in the brain rise. If the brain swells, the body attempts to compensate by reducing cerebral blood flow or production of cerebral spinal fluid. When the body is unable to compensate for the abnormal pressures, the pressures moves the brain tissue down through the foramen magnum. The foramen magnum is the bony opening at the base of the skull.

NEUROLOGY 12 answers

1. Explain the difference between an embolic stroke versus a hemorrhagic stroke.
   An embolic stroke (also called an ischemic stroke) occurs when the blood flow is impeded. A hemorrhagic stroke occurs when a blood vessel ruptures resulting in bleeding into the brain.
2. What does hypercapnia cause in the brain?
   Hypercapnia increases blood flow to the brain. When the brain has injury or a hemorrhage, this can increase brain edema further causing more damage.
3. What happens in the brain when the patient is hyperventilated.

Hyperventilation results in cerebral vasoconstriction. This will prevent adequate blood flow to the brain reduced oxygenation to the brain.

4. Why are stool softeners ordered for patients with a head injury. Explain how intracranial pressure plays a role.
   Constipation may cause the patient to bear down thus increasing intra-abdominal pressure. Intra-abdominal pressure can cause an increase in intracranial pressures.
5. Explain the physiological differences between the following and their significance.

Decorticate posturing	The arms are flexed toward the center of the body with the wrist flexed and the hands curled. The legs are rigid with pointed toes.
Decerebrate posturing	The arms are extended with the flexed wrist and curled fingers. The legs are rigid and the toes pointed.

6. Explain the difference between the following

Diabetes insipidus	The patient voids copious amount of urine thus ridding the body of fluids
Syndrome of inappropriate antidiuretic syndrome.	The patient retains fluids.

NEUROLOGY 13 answers

1. Match the following

Hemorrhagic stroke	Clot traveled from the body to cerebral artery
Thrombotic stroke	Arterial rupture
Embolic stroke	Occlusion from an accumulation of platelets and fibrin on an atherosclerotic plaque

(Hemorrhagic stroke → Arterial rupture; Thrombotic stroke → Occlusion from an accumulation of platelets and fibrin on an atherosclerotic plaque; Embolic stroke → Clot traveled from the body to cerebral artery)

2. List two neurological issues that may occur in a patient with a right hemispheric stroke.
Vision and hearing problems. May have problems with balance.

3. Define, what is neurogenic shock?

A condition that may affect vital signs due to damage to the nervous system. Neurogenic shock results in hemodynamic changes.

3. Define the following:

Orthostatic hypotension	Low blood pressure that occurs when rising from sitting or lying
Autonomic dysreflexia	Abnormal over-reaction of the autonomic nervous system due to painful sensory input
laminectomy	A surgical procedure to remove a portion of the vertebra to remove a herniated disc or the pressure on a compressed nerve.

4. Explain the relationship between sensation and dermatomes.

The dermatomes are nerve roots that relay sensation from a particular area of the body. There are 30 pairs of spinal nerves. Each dermatome has a designated area of sensation.

NEUROLOGY 14 answers

1. Match the following

Hemorrhagic stroke	Clot traveled from the body to cerebral artery
Thrombotic stroke	Arterial rupture
Embolic stroke	Occlusion from an accumulation of platelets and fibrin on an atherosclerotic plaque

Hemorrhagic stroke → Arterial rupture
Thrombotic stroke → Occlusion from an accumulation of platelets and fibrin on an atherosclerotic plaque
Embolic stroke → Clot traveled from the body to cerebral artery

2. List two neurological issues that may occur in a patient with a right hemispheric stroke.
   Vision and hearing problems. May have problems with balance.

3. Define, what is neurogenic shock?

> A condition that may affect vital signs due to damage to the nervous system. Neurogenic shock results in hemodynamic changes.

4. Define the following:

Orthostatic hypotension	Low blood pressure that occurs when rising from sitting or lying
Autonomic dysreflexia	Abnormal over-reaction of the autonomic nervous system due to painful sensory input
laminectomy	A surgical procedure to remove a portion of the vertebra to remove a herniated disc or the pressure on a compressed nerve.

5. Explain the relationship between sensation and dermatomes.

> The dermatomes are nerve roots that relay sensation from a particular area of the body. There are 30 pairs of spinal nerves. Each dermatome has a designated area of sensation.

NEUROLOGY 15 answers

Match the following

1. Contusion	A. A blood leak
2. Hematoma	B. Bruises on the parenchyma
3. Epidural hematoma	C. Blood between the skull and the dura mater
4. Subdural hematoma	D. Bleeding between the arachnoid and the pia mater
5. Subarachnoid hemorrhage	E. Collection of blood
6. Intracranial hemorrhage	F. Blood between the dura mater and the arachnoid layer

1. __B____ 2. ___E____ 3. ___C____ 4. ___F____ 5. ___D____ 6. __A____

List what may be included in a bedside neurological assessment. (remember to include vital signs)

> Patient's level of consciousness, level of awareness, orientation, and motor responses. PERRLA. Vital signs. Sensation assessment. Cranial nerve assessment. Assessment of reflexes. Ability to speak, understand, and swallow.

1. What is a pronator drift? A pathological test in a neurological assessment which will indicate muscle weakness or abnormal function.

2. What is the rationale for frequent cranial nerve and pupil assessments in the patient with a head injury. Changes that may occur in the cranial nerves response to testing may be indicative of a declining or worse condition.

Define the following and why it is assessed.

3. Corneal reflex: The corneal reflex can determine if there are issues with the trigeminal and facial cranial nerves. IF there are issues with the corneal reflex, it can indicate brain stem lesion, brain stem stroke, or Parkinson's disease. This test cranial nerve 5 & 7.

4. Cough reflex: The cough reflex is a protective mechanism that is stimulated when the respiratory tract is irritated by dust or foreign particles. The cough reflex is assessed to test the Vagus nerve.

5. Gag reflex: The protective reaction of the body to protect the airway. It is assessed to ensure the patient can protect their airway. This tests cranial nerve 9 & 10.

6. Babinski reflex: A test to assess the plantar reflex. It assists to evaluate a neurological issue in an adult or a patient older that two years of age.

NEUROLOGY 16 answers

Briefly define the following test/procedure

1. Neurological imaging: Medical imaging (CT scan or MRI) that indirectly or directly produce images of the structures of the brain to investigate the brain structures, physiology and function.

2. Intracranial monitoring: The inserting of a device into the head to monitor the pressures inside the skull.

3. Cerebral blood flow: Cerebral blood flow also known as a perfusion study, measures the rate of arterial blood passing through the brain tissue.

4. C.T. scan: A computed tomography is a test using an x-ray like image with computer technology to produce detailed images of the ordered body part.

5. M.R. I.: Magnetic resonance imaging is an imaging test that creates images by using a large magnet and radio waves.

6. Angiography: An angiography is an X-ray that which the use of contrast can visualize the blood vessels.

Answer the following:

7. What is the difference between a subarachnoid bolt and an ICP drain? A subarachnoid bolt is inserted into the brain but only allows intracranial pressure monitor. An intracranial pressure drain allows monitoring as well as drainage of cerebral spinal fluid.

8. What is a transcranial doppler ultrasonography? A transcranial doppler (TCD) ultrasound uses sound waves to detect abnormalities that affect blood flow in the brain (blood clots, hemorrhage, or vasospasms).

9. What is an electrophysiologic monitoring (EEG)? Give an example when it would be used. An EEG an external device that measures the electrical activity of the brain. It is often used in seizure patients to determine the seizure activity or abnormal electrical paths in the brain.

10. What is the end goal in the treatment of the patient with a head injury? The end goal is to prevent a decline in brain injury by the use of monitoring equipment, controlling hemorrhaging, maintaining adequate oxygenation and monitoring the vital signs.

11. What is a transtentorial herniation? A transtentorial herniation is when the brain tissue moves from one area (compartment) to another.

12. Why should the nurse not attempt to place a nasogastric tube in the patient with a basilar skull fracture? The Cribriform plate is a thin bone at the end of the nasal cavity which can be fractured in the patient with a head injury. When attempting to insert the nasogastric tube, the tube could slide through the fractured bone into the brain.

13. Why should hypotonic IV fluids be avoided in the patient with a head injury? Hypotonic fluids shift into the tissues which increase edema. In the patient with a brain injury, this fluid can cause worsening cerebral edema.

14. When is ICP monitoring considered appropriate? When a patient is determined to have a Glasgow Coma scale score below 8 or when imaging reflects abnormality.

15. What does it mean if the patient is posturing? Posturing occurs in the patients with severe damage to the brain or abnormal brain activity.

16. Why should hypercapnia be monitored in the patient with a head injury? Abnormal levels of hypercapnia can increase brain swelling.

17. What occurs when a patient with a traumatic brain injury is hyperventilated? Hyperventilation will cause cerebral vasoconstriction.

18. List three medications that maybe used to control intracranial pressure.

a. Mannitol (an osmotic diuretic)

b. Furosemide (a loop diuretic)

c. Decadron (dexamethasone) is a corticosteroid.

NEUROLOGY 17 answers

1. Why should the nurse enforce a low or no stimulation for the traumatic brain injured patient? To avoid overstimulation. Overstimulation of the patient with a traumatic brain injury (TBI) can increase intracranial pressures.

2. The patient with a traumatic head injury has been hyperthermic then hypothermic without any intervention. Explain why this occurs. The brain injured patient may have injuries or swelling to the hypothalamus (regulates body temperature). This fluctuation is not caused by an infectious source. Patients with fluctuation temperatures after a traumatic brain injury have poor prognosis.

3. Why must the nurse monitor for the following in the neurologically injured patient?

    d. Vasospasms: Preventing vasospasms or the treatment of vasospasms can assist to prevent permanent neurological deficits.

    e. Seizures: seizures can impact the brain by causing hypoperfusion or brain hypoxia.

    f. Intracranial infections: Monitoring for intracranial infections can assist to identify a potential secondary brain injury.

4. Why are anticonvulsants prophylactically prescribed for the traumatic brain injured patient? Anticonvulsants are prophylactically used in the traumatic brain injured patient to prevent early post-trauma seizures. Seizures may result in a secondary brain injury.

5. What are trickle feeds and why are they an important part in the nutritional support in the patient with a traumatic brain injured patient? Head injuries increase the metabolic needs for the body. Trickle feeds begin the nutritional replacement needs. Trickle feeds are liquid food (tube feeding) that is given to the patient via a nasogastric tube, or percutaneous esophagogastrostomy tube (PEG). Calories can also be given via IV if tube feedings.

Often the nurse must use the following to assess the response of the neurologically injured patient. Briefly describe the following and what it means if there is or isn't a response.

a. Trapezius pinch: Pinching 2 inches (thick muscle) to elicit a response to assess the level of consciousness of the patient.

b. Nail bed pressure: Pressure is applied to the nail to achieve a response to assess the level of consciousness of the patient.

1. List two interventions that a nurse may use to reduce a brain injured patient's ICP.

    Raise the head of the bed (if not contraindicated by a spinal injury), keep the neck in a neutral position, keep a quiet environment, and keep a reduced light environment.

2. What are battle signs? Battle signs are bruising over the mastoid process that indicates a fracture at the base of the skull.

3. What are racoon eyes? Periorbital ecchymosis or bilateral dark purple or bluish colored bruises under the eyes.

4. Which part of the brain has the respiratory control center? The medulla oblongata (in the lower brain stem) regulates breathing.

NINE PROVISIONS OF THE NURSING CODE OF ETHICS answers

List each provision and give an example of a nursing action or intervention for each.

1. Provision 1: The nurse practices with compassion and respect for the inherent dignity, worth, and unique attributes of every person.
   Example: Provide for privacy when assessing the patient.
2. Provision 2: The nurse's primary commitment is to the patient, whether individual, family, groups, community, or population.
   Example: The nurse in the advocate role.
3. Provision 3: The nurse promotes, advocates for, and protects the rights, health, and safety of the patient.
   Example: The patient does not want a blood transfusion but will not survive without the blood. The nurse will advocate for the patient's wishes.
4. Provision 4: The nurse has authority, accountability, and responsibility for nursing practice: makes decisions, and takes action consistent with the obligation to promote health and to provide optimal care.
   Example: The patient may choose to consult the case manager to ensure the patient has home health care assistance until the patient fully recovers.
5. Provision 5: The nurse owes the same duties to self as to others, including the responsibility to preserve integrity and safety, to maintain competence, and to continue personal and professional growth.
   Examples: The nurse makes certain to take scheduled days off, eat well, and rest.
6. Provision 6: The nurse, through individual and collective effort, establishes, maintains, and improves the ethical environment of the work setting and conditions of employment that are conducive to safe, quality health care.
   Example: The nurse may need to report unsafe staffing ratios.
7. Provision 7: All nurses engage in scholarly activity by providing evidence-informed practice. Nurse researchers follow national-international standards for conducting research with human participants. All research must be approved by institutional review boards (IRBs) in compliance with national standards.
   Example: the nurse ensures to incorporate best practices in their nursing practice.
8. Provision 8: The nurse collaborates with other health professionals and the public to protect human rights, promote health diplomacy, and reduce health disparities.
   Example: The nurse includes self in the interdisciplinary team.
9. Provision 9: The profession of nursing, collectively through its professional organizations, must articulate nursing values, maintain the integrity of the profession, and integrate principles of social justice into nursing and health policy.
   Example: Join a nursing association
A. Define ethics.: The rational justification of what is right and wrong.
B. Name two ethical issues nurses face today. Explain your response. Resource allocation and opioid crisis. Resources may be low and determining who should receive those resources is an

ethical dilemma. When Covid-19 occurred, ventilators may have been given to those patients who were deemed more likely to recover. The opioid crisis may prevent a healthcare facility from prescribing appropriate pain medication for fear of patient addiction or repercussions from state monitoring agencies.

C. What is the ethics committee and what is their role in an ethical family conflict? A ethics committee is an independent healthcare body composed of members with various backgrounds and expertise. The committee attempts to resolve ethical dilemmas through family meetings.

D. Define advocacy and give an example of an ethical situation that you may face as a nurse. Advocacy is the action taken by the nurse to plead on behalf of the patient. The patient may wish to die instead of continuing treatment. The doctors may not agree with the patient's choice.

E. How does autonomy, justice, beneficence, and nonmaleficence play a role in ethics? Autonomy is allowing the patient to make their own decision. Justice is assuring a fair decision. Beneficence is doing good, such as supporting the patient's choice. Nonmaleficence is ensuring no harm while supporting the patient's choice.

F. Explain how the nurse's ethical decision may play a role in employer backlash. The nurse may report a nursing shortage which places patient's safety at risk. The manager may not want to spend the extra money to hire more staff. The nurse may report this situation to the state board. The health care system could be fined. The manager may make work life uncomfortable for the nurse. The nurse may need to decide how to handle this situation. Stay and attempt to improve the work place environment or quit and work elsewhere.

G. Explain the relationship between ethics and research. Research involves the principles of ethics. The participants must be given their rights, and notification of their choice to quit at any time. This must be in the consent.

NURSING HISTORY answers

Match the nurse to the accomplishment

1.	Clarissa (Clara) Barton
2.	Mary Breckinridge
3.	Virginia Henderson
4.	Hazel W. Johnson-Brown
5.	Mary Eliza Mahoney
6.	Florence Nightingale
7.	Margaret Sanger
8.	Sojourner Truth
9.	Dorothea Dix
10.	Anna Caroline Maxwell
11.	Lillian Ward
12.	Jacqueline Fawcett

a. Organized first army nurse corps
b. Founder of American Birth control league which later became planned parenthood
c. Co-founder of the National Association of Colored graduate nurses
d. Activist-advocated for nurse education for African-American nurses
e. Founded first science-based nursing school
f. Founded the Red Cross of America
g. Founded frontier nursing & midwifery

h. Theorist. Shaped nursing education with the nursing need theory
i. Director of Walter Reed. First Afro-American woman general
j. Advocate for better treatment of the mentally ill
k. Pioneered public health nursing in U.S.
l. Expert in nursing conceptual models & theories.

Answer section

1. ___F_____
2. ____G_____
3. ____H_____
4. ____i____
5. ____C_____
6. ____E_____
7. ____B_____
8. ____D_____
9. ___J_____
10. ____A____
11. ___K_____
12. ____L____

NURSING PROCESS 1 answers

1. What is the purpose of the nursing assessment? To gather data about the patient's overall health and current concerns.

2. List three assessment skills needed to perform a thorough assessment. Inspection, palpitation, percussion and auscultation

3. What is subjective data? Information collected from the patient or the patient's family.

4. What is objective data? Factual data that can be observed or measured.

5. List 2 sources in which subjective data can be collected. The patient and the patient's family.

6. What can be done if there are discrepancies in the subjective data collected? Critical thinking skills will assist to deduce the correct data.

7. What is intuition and how does it play a role in assessment? Intuition is a feeling. Nurses often have intuition that assists them to make better judgements.

8. What method is used to organize the data collected by the nurse? Nurses use interviews, therapeutic communication, focus, clustering data, and analysis.

9. How does clustering data aid the nurse in determining priority problems? Clustering data will assist to identify priority problems by identifying problems in a systematic way.

10. What is an initial assessment? A thorough assessment completed on the admission of a patient.

11. What is a focused assessment? An assessment that focuses on the patient's current health issue.

12. Should an initial assessment be completed each shift? Explain your response. An initial assessment is completed when the patient is admitted. A shift assessment is completed thereafter.

13. Should a holistic assessment be part of the initial assessment or only focused on the patient? Explain your response. The holistic assessment should be part of the initial assessment. The assessment is focused on the whole patient and not simply focuses on the current health issue.

14. What type of assessment must be completed in an emergent situation? In an emergent situation, the patient should be assessed in a systematic way. Airway, breathing, circulation, disability, and exposure.

15. What is a concept map? A concept map is a visual map of information that can be organized to determine the priority problems.

16. How does a concept map guide the student? A concept map assists the student to determine the relationship of the collected data.

17. What is a nursing care plan? A nursing care plan lays out the planned goals, interventions to achieve those goals, and the evaluation of these efforts.

18. Is a nursing care plan prepared solely for the use of nurses caring for the patient? Explain your response. Everyone on the patient's healthcare team use the plan of care prepared by the nurse. The physicians, nursing assistants, respiratory therapist, physical therapy, and the nurse.

NURSING WORKSHEET 1 answers

1. Explain the difference between dereliction of duty and abandonment in nursing. Give an example of each. Dereliction of duty is failure to perform an obligation. Failing to give medications. Abandonment is permanently leaving the patient. Walking out on the assignment.

2. Should a nursing student or a nurse have malpractice insurance? Explain the pros and cons of having malpractice insurance. Yes. Incidents happen and patients sue. It is better to be protected and have peace of mind. The cons of having malpractice insurance is that a premium must be paid annually.

3. A patient or the patient's family may have unrealistic expectations of the care and treatment of the patient. "We saw on the internet this new herbal medication that stops cancer, cures diabetes, and reverses heart failure. Can't you try that?" Explain the response you would give. The internet is not an accurate and valid source of data. Only researched facts with confirmed outcomes should be considered. Also, information on the internet may be old and obsolete.

4. Define documentation. Documentation serves as a record and a timeline of events. It is data that is entered on a timely manner on the tasks provided, response of those tasks, and current health data such as vital signs and laboratory results.

5. When must the nurse or other healthcare team members document in the patient's chart? Documentation should be completed in a timely manner. This will allow any of the interdisciplinary team members to view any updates that may impact their role in care.

6. When is it acceptable to document at the end of the shift? (Think emergent situations). If the nurse is needed at the bedside due to a patient's declining health status, the nurse's focus should be on the care of the patient and then document at the end of the shift or when the patient is stable.

7. You are asked to work in the emergency room. A patient is admitted by ambulance. The patient is in respiratory distress, unconscious, and without family or friend. The doctor orders oxygen, a breathing treatment, and a steroid. Can you administer the steroid without knowing any past medical history or allergy status of the patient? Explain your answer. Yes. Care of the patient must be done due to the emergent health situation. If the patient is unable to offer allergy information and lack of family or friend, treatment should not be held as it could be lethal.

8. You are driving home. You see a car accident with the driver pinned behind the wheel. You rush to help. The patient is unconscious. The gas tank has ruptured and the hot motor may ignite the gas at any time. You remove the driver and drag him yards away moments before the car erupts into flame. The patient is later diagnosed with spinal injuries resulting in paralysis due to being removed from the car without a cervical collar or spine support. Explain how the Good

Samaritan law will protect you. The good Samaritan law offers legal protection to people who assist those who are injured or in peril.

9. A patient that was angry with the doctor is discharged. Four years later the patient decides he will sue. Explain what statue of limitations is and does it apply to this scenario. Explain your response. It depends on the state on the limitations. However; most malpractice lawsuit limitations is 2 to 5 years or 3 years from the when the patient should have known the causation for the lawsuit.

10. What is administrative law and how does it differ from rules and regulations set forth by the state? Administrative law is determined by state and federal governmental agencies and administrative law incorporates policies that fall within the governmental law.

PAIN 1 answers

1. Match the following

WORD	DEFINITION
1. Modulation	a. Converts painful stimuli to an electrical impulse
2. Transduction	b. The point at which a person feels pain
3. Transmission	c. Move away from a painful stimulus
4. Threshold	d. Traveling of impulses that reduce the intensity of the stimulus
5. Tolerance	e. Level in which the person is willing and able to handle

1. __D__ 2. __A__ 3. __C__ 4. __B__ 5. __E__

2. Match the following.

1. Acute pain	a. Recurrent. Last greater than six months.
2. Chronic pain	b. Pain from damaged nerves
3. Nociceptive pain	c. Sudden onset. Temporary. Last less than six months. Usually resolves
4. Neuropathic pain	d. Pain from damage to or inflammation of tissue(s)

1. __C__ 2. __A__ 3. __D__ 4. __B__

2. List causes of the following.

Chronic pain	Acute pain
Arthritis	Surgical intervention
Back pain	A broken arm
neuropathy	A gunshot

PAIN 2 answers

1. List ways to manage pain. List pharmacological and non-pharmacological methods.

Pharmacological methods	Non-pharmacological methods
IV pain medications	Back rub
Oral over-the-counter pain relievers	Warm bath or shower
Opioid medication	Heating pad
Muscle relaxers	Ice pack
Corticosteroids	Proper alignment of the body or part
Antidepressants	Soft music
Topical pain ointment	meditation
Antiseizure medication	Scent therapy

2. List what data a nurse may ask a patient regarding the patient's pain.

   What happened. When did it happen. Location of pain. Describe the character of the pain. Intensity of the pain. Duration of the pain. Did anything help relieve the pain? What aggravates the pain? What makes the pain worse?

3. List three types of nociceptive pain.
   Superficial
   Somatic
   Visceral

4. What is COX1 and COX2? How do they differ and how are they similar? (Cyclooxygenases)
   COX1 and COX2 are key enzymes that assist in the production of prostaglandins. COX1 is mainly involved in the protective processes of the body. COX2 is involved in the inflammatory processes of the body.

5. How do prostaglandins play a role in pain? There are different types of prostaglandins. Some may suppress inflammation, some may cause inflammation, while others may be involved in blood clotting or bleeding.

PAIN 3 answers

1. When assessing pain, what does intensity refer to? Pain intensity refers to the magnitude of pain.

2. How would you assess the quality of the patient's pain? What does quality mean? To assess the quality of pain, the nurse would use a pain scale. For adults, the numeric pain scale is used. Quality is used to ask to describe the pain. How it feels to the patient.

3. What is a FLACC pain scale? A pain scale used for non-verbal patients using behavioral cues. Example: groaning, guarding, or elevated blood pressure.

4. On what type of patient's would the FLACC pain scale be used? A patient who had a cerebral vascular accident and aphagia or an intubated patient on a ventilator.

5. List two barriers to effective pain management. Provider interpretation of the pain scale and the experienced pain by the patient. Cultural attitudes. Provider attitudes toward the type of patient (example: street drug abuser).

6. Define the following pain scales and on which patient population it would be used.

SCALE	DEFINE/POPULATION
NIPS	Behavioral pain scale used for newborn babies
WONG-BAKER	A face pain scale. It shows a smiling face (no pain) to a crying face (10 pain level). This scale is used for children
CRIES	A pain scale used to measure pain in a neonate.
FLACC	The FLACC scale is a behavioral scale used for 2 months to 7 years or nonverbal patients
NUMBER	A pain scale for adults. Measures pain from zero (no pain) to 10 (worse pain)
BEHAVIORAL	Used for pain in the unconscious or intubated patient

7. Why is so difficult to manage pain in a patient with a substance abuse problem? The substance abuser has built up a tolerance to pain medications.

8. What is meant by a comprehensive pain assessment? Exploring various areas of pain. Evaluating what the person is feeling experiencing the pain, how it may have an impact on the patient's life (financially or physically such as ADL or in their relationship), and how it impacts sleep.

9. What is a common physical complication of narcotic usage? Sedation, respiratory depression, nausea, vomiting, constipation, tolerance, and addiction.

10. Can pain be controlled completely? Explain your response. Not all pain can be controlled completely. It maybe managed to a level of tolerance (a level the patient can live with).

PAIN 4 answers

1. What is epidural pain management and what does it target? Epidural pain management uses a catheter inserted into the epidural space to numb spinal nerves that block pain in a specific area of the body.

2. What are the benefits of epidural pain management? It provides pain relief in situations that normally would require anesthesia. Such as during child birth or surgery.

3. What concerns or side effects may occur with epidural pain management? Hypotension, headaches, or pruritus.

4. What is the difference between acute pain and chronic pain? Acute pain is sudden onset that can last less than 3 months. Chronic pain can last 3 months or greater.

5. How can pain be assessed and managed in the non-verbal patient? By using a behavioral pain scale to assessment the patient prior to medication administration. Then use the behavioral pain scale to reassess the effectiveness of the pain medication one hour later.

6. Is there a difference between opioid dependence and addiction? Explain your response. A person can become physically dependent on the opioids without becoming addicted. An example is someone with severe arthritis. They physically depend on the opioid but are not addicted to the opioid.

7. What is complex regional pain syndrome? Complex regional pain syndrome is chronic pain of an extremity that developed due to a health issue (CVA) or surgical intervention.

8. Explain how untreated pain may affect the immune system. Pain increases the cortisol levels which results in decreased function of the body's immune system.

PAIN 5 answers

1. Why shouldn't the patient be given unrealistic pain control expectations? Patients that are given unrealistic pain control expectations can become unsatisfied with their care. Communication on patient expectations and what is the reality of the situation can aid in patient satisfaction

2. List five behaviors that may indicate pain.

1.	Moaning
2.	Body guarding or thrashing in bed
3.	High blood pressure
4.	High heart rate
5.	High respiratory rate

3. Explain how a pain scale can be objectively used to assess pain. Comparing the patient's response to behavioral pain indicators

4. Can pain be assessed in the intubated pain? Explain your response. Pain can be assessed by using a behavioral pain scale. It uses vital signs and body movements to assess pain.

5. Why is it difficult to assess pain in the patient with a history of drug abuse? The patient may be drug seeking. The patient may have been abusing opioids which can result in a low pain tolerance.

6. What is an opioid risk tool and why or when should it be used? An opioid risk tool is a screening tool used to accurately predict opioid use of the patient and potential addiction. It should be used for every patient who may be prescribed an opioid and are at risk of addiction or those who suffer from chronic pain.

7. What is an analgesic ladder? A guide for prescribing pain management drugs.

8. What is considered mild pain? Pain that can be treated with nonopioid medications

9. What is considered moderate pain? Pain that can be treated with either a nonopioid medication as well as a therapy (whirlpool, heating pad, ice pack) and a weak opioid medication

10. What is considered severe pain? Pain that requires a strong opioid along with a nonopioid and therapy

11. List four factors that play a role in determining drug addiction.

Peer pressure
Stress
Physical and/or sexual abuse
Risky behavior

PAIN 6 answers

1. Explain how opioids bind to mu, kappa, and delta sites. Mu, kappa, and delta are opioid binding sites that mediate the body's response to drugs. These sites play a central role in nociception and analgesia. Each site has an area of the brain in which it is more effective. Opioids are agonist that stimulate Mu, Kappa, and delta.

2. Can genetic variability affect opioid effectiveness? Explain your response. Yes. Genetic variation may directly affect opioids absorption and metabolism. How the phenotype responses to opioids is a result of genetics.

3. What is intrathecal pain control? Intrathecal pain control is infusing medication directly into the spinal cord through a surgically implanted device.

4. What is a nerve block? A nerve block is an injection into the nerve area to treat pain.

5. What is a Q-pump? A fixed flow pump that continuously delivers a local anesthesia to a patient's surgical site.

6. What is a PCA? A patient controlled analgesia pump is a infusion pump specific for medication that allows the patient to self-deliver pain medications per the physicians orders.

7. Why is there a concern for the PCA by proxy? A proxy may give the patient too much pain medication or too little. It is safer for the patient to be the sole user of the PCA.

8. Briefly explain what a multimodal analgesic regime is and why it can enhance pain relief. Multimodal analgesic regime uses non-narcotic with narcotic medication to enhance pain relief. An example of multimodal analgesia is when administering Tylenol with codeine. It can enhance pain relief.

9. What is a narcotic? A narcotic is a pain medication that bind to opioid receptors and assist to control pain.

10. How should narcotics be disposed? In the hospital, place in the black box. Outside the hospital, you can take to a pharmacy.

11. When a narcotic is ordered, why should the lowest dose be given instead of the highest dose? Pain medication is often prescribed by a pain scale. More pain medication may be given if the pain is not relieved. If too much is given, it places the patient's health in jeopardy.

12. List two medications that may potentiate the effectiveness of a narcotic. Phenytoin, Carbamazepine, or phenobarbital.

13. List two medications that may considered antagonist of a narcotic. Naloxone and naltrexone.

14. What does it mean to potentiate? To increase effect

15. What does it mean to be an antagonist medication? A substance that halts the effect of a medication.

16. List three other interventions that may assist with pain relief in conjunction with the administration of the pain medication. Heating pad. Ice pack. Massage. Music. Acupuncture.

17. List two narcotics that may be given in oral, intramuscular, and IV form. Morphine and Fentanyl.

18. How long does it take an intramuscular pain medication to begin working? It depends on the medication but the usual time is 10 – 30 minutes.

PAIN SCALES answers

Match the following pain scale with their description

Pain tool	Description	Correct match
I. Numeric scale	9. Used in critical care areas to assess pain based on observation	i. 3
J. N-Pass scale	10. Assessment for advanced dementia patients	j. 8
K. FLACC scale	11. (9 year old to elderly) Assessed via perceived level of pain	k. 5
L. FACES scale	12. Observational tool used for critical care	l. 6
M. CRIES scale	13. (Infant to 7 years) observation based tool	m. 7
N. Behavioral scale	14. Wong-Baker scale for 3 years (plus)	n. 4
O. CPOT scale	15. Scale for babies 8 months to 16 months	o. 1
P. PAINAD	16. Scale used for neonates	p. 2

Mark the behaviors that maybe observed in the cognitively impaired patient experiencing pain.

- Moaning
- Guarding
- Thrashing
- **Sleeping calmly**
- **Shallow respirations**
- Frequent moving

PARKINSON'S DISEASE ANSWERS

A 73 year-old man is admitted with a diagnosis of Parkinson's disease. Choose from the following, which, if any, are used to diagnose

	Used to diagnose P.D.
EMG & NCV	
Anti-acetylcholine receptor antibody test	
PMH & Symptoms	X
MRI	

Answer information:

Parkinson's disease is diagnosed from past medical history and presented symptoms. EMG & NCV, and the Anti-acetylcholine receptor antibody test is used to diagnose myasthenia Gravis. An MRI is used to diagnose multiple sclerosis

The nurse knows there are classical symptoms of Parkinson's disease, known as the triad of P.D. Choose from the list below those symptoms.

	Symptom of Parkinson's disease
Rigidity	X
Ptosis	
Lhermitte's sign	
Bradykinesia	X
Tremors at rest	X
Muscle wasting	
Restless leg syndrome	

Answer information:

Ptosis & restless leg syndrome are symptoms in Myasthenia Gravis (MG).

Lhermitte sign is a symptom in multiple sclerosis (MS).

Muscle wasting is seen in ALS, MG, and MS.

Which of the following is the initial sign of Parkinson's disease

	Initial sign
Cognitive wheel rigidity	
Festination (shuffling gait)	
Pill rolling	X
Masked face	

Answer information:

All signs of Parkinson's disease. Pill rolling (tremors) are the first sign of Parkinson's disease.

The doctor orders diphenhydramine (Benadryl) for the Parkinson's disease patient. You anticipate this medication is ordered to:

	Answer
Control allergies	
Manage tremors	X
Assist to sleep	
Rash	

Answer information:

Diphenhydramine has anticholinergic properties and therefore can assist to manage tremors.

As a nurse, you recognize nutrition management is important. Choose which of the following is not a good nutritional choice for the patient taking Levodopa.

	Answer
Provide adequate roughage	
Provide fortified cereals	X
Provide cut food into small bite size pieces	
Provide 6 small meals daily	

Answer information:

Fortified cereal contain vitamin B6 which impairs absorption of Levodopa.

Which of the following does not result in drug(s) induced Parkinson's disease.

	Answer
Methyldopa	
Propranolol	X
Lithium	
Haloperidol	
chlorpromazine	

Answer information:

Propranolol is a B-adrenergic blocker and is often used to treat tremors in Parkinson patients.

Methyldopa, lithium, haloperidol, and chlorpromazine as well as Illicit drugs can cause drug induced Parkinson's disease

The doctor discusses a deep-brain stimulator (DBS). Choose which of the following area that is not considered for electrode placement.

	Answer
Thalamus	
Lateral Corticospinal tract	X
Subthalmic nucleus	
Globus pallidus	

Answer information:

The lateral corticospinal tract contains fibers that descends down the spine to control voluntary movements of limbs on the opposite side of its tract.

PATIENT CARE 1 answers

1. The nurse must promote a supportive and safe environment. Patients often fear their pain will not be addressed effectively. List ways the nurse can ensure the patient's pain is assessed and pain control measures are implemented. (Include patient education.) Explain to the patient, once pain medication is administered, the patient will be reassessed in one hour for effectiveness. The patient can be notified when the next dose is available. The patient should be educated to notify the nurse if the medication is not effective. The patient may need a different medication.

2. Explain how trust plays a key role in patient education. Communicating with the patient and keeping the patient informed of all expectations will assist to build trust.

3. Pain is considered the sixth vital sign. List the various types of pain scales available. Give an example of what type or age of the patient the nurse would use for each pain scale.

    Number pain scale: adults
    FACE pain scale: children
    FLACC pain scale: infants 0 – 12 months
    Behavioral scale: Non-verbal patients (adult or children)

4. When assessing pain, what data would the nurse need to know prior to calling the doctor for a pain medication? How it happened. Duration. Character. Location. What makes it worse. What makes it better. Has it occurred before? What medications usually work for pain.

5. Explain why it is important to know the patient's previous medical history. The patient may have a condition that may affect treatment. Allergies. Medications that may not be compatible with what may be used for the current condition. The patient may have substance abuse issues.

6. Why is it important to complete a head-to-toe assessment on a patient within 24 hours of admission? In the event a change occurs with the patient, it can be compared with the initial assessment. An example would be if the patient developed a pressure ulcer.

7. What is the importance of assessing the patient's skin daily? To ensure there are no breakdowns. Precautions can be taken if the skin appears to be compromised.

8. Explain the necessity of reading the previous nurses notes. The patient may have a significant change that warrants notifying the doctor. For example, if the patient's blood pressure is usually 150/80 and the current reading is 90/40 and the patient was admitted for gastrointestinal bleed, this may indicate a severe hemorrhage.

9. When should patient education begin? Explain your answer. Patient education should begin at the time of admission and continue throughout the hospitalization. The patient should be educated to the hospital routine, medications, orders, allowed activities, visiting hours, etc. The doctor will notify the patient of health needs, such as laboratory test, CT scans, surgery, etc.

10. What is the best way to assess the patient's genitals without embarring the patient? Explain you need to assess the femoral pulses and view while taking the pulse. The nurse can assess when the patient has the patient turned on their side and view from the back.

11. Can the patient refuse to be assessed? Explain your answer. Yes. The patient must be informed that by refusing, they (the patient) takes the responsibility for any complications that occur as a result of the refusal. Often the doctor, once notified, will inform the patient if they do not cooperate, they will be discharge. Since the purpose of a hospitalization is to be carefully monitored.

12. Why is it important to orient the patient to the room? The patient needs to know where the call bell, room lights, and telephone may be. They may also need to be instructed to remain in bed until the nurse or Patient care technician comes into the room before attempting to get out of bed.

13. Your patient decides he doesn't want to stay in the hospital. You know he needs more medical care. Does your patient have the right to leave? Explain your answer. Yes. It is called AMA. Against medical advice. The patient must sign a paper stating the responsibility of leaving falls on them for choosing to leave before medically cleared to do so.

14. What does AMA stand for? Against medical advice.

PATIENT CARE WORKSHEET 2 answers

1. You are working in the emergency room. A child is brought in with an elevated temperature. You notice a lot of bruises on the child. Do you need to explain to the parents that you need to make out a report for child abuse? Explain your answer. No. All healthcare providers are mandated to report any suspicion of abuse or neglect.

2. List the signs that may present in a patient that has been abused. Bruises, multiple broken bones, weight loss, old clothing, unkempt, odorous, the patient may be frightful and assume a fetal or protective posture.

3. List the signs that may be present in a patient that is neglected. Dirty. Odorous. old clothing. Malnourished. Dehydrated. Long nails.

4. Your shift in the emergency room has not ended. An adolescent comes in and requests treatment for venereal disease. Can you treat this patient or do you require parental consent? Explain your answer. Yes. This patient can be treated without parental consent. However; it is always best practice to check with the local health department.

5. You are assigned a suicidal adolescent who is having difficulty in breathing. He doesn't want any medical intervention. He says, "I just want to die. Leave me alone." What interventions, if any, would you do? The patient is depressed and cannot be allowed to make decisions that will result in his death. He needs to be treated and seen by a psychiatrist to ensure adequate follow through on his suicidal wishes.

6. The doctor wants your suicidal adolescent admitted to the mental health ward. The patient is refusing. Describe how you would explain the difference between voluntary and involuntary commitment to your patient. A voluntary commitment is an agreement with the patient that they agree to admission to the mental health unit for a minimum (usually 3 days) allotted time frame. Involuntary is when the patient is petitioned to be placed in the mental health unit until the doctor believes the patient is fit to be discharged.

7. What is the difference between a chronic disease and an acute disease. Include an example of each. An acute disease has a sudden onset and last for a short period of time. An example of an acute disease is a broken arm. A chronic disease is a condition that last for a duration of 3 months or longer. An example of a chronic disease is arthritis.

8. You have been assigned as a preceptor for a new nurse. Explain how you will teach critical judgement. Practice critical decisions with scenarios. Use reasoning skills. Take time to reflect on the situation before making a decision.

9. What is good faith reporting? Good faith reporting is when the nurse suspects abuse and reports the abuse to authorities.

10. Your orientee has made a medication error. What should you do? Explain your response. Write the medication error on the hospital incident form. Tell the charge nurse. Inform the doctor and the patient.

11. Nosocomial infections are always waiting to happen. What can you, as a health care professional do to help prevent the spread of a nosocomial infection? Wash hands between patients and when entering or leaving each patient room. Never use equipment without first cleaning the equipment if previously used (example- bladder scanner). Follow protocols on isolation patients.

12. Your orientee asks you, "What is evidence-based-practice?" How will you respond? Evidence-based practice (EBP) is applying research findings that have been proved to improve patient care into your nursing practice.

PATIENT CARE WORKSHEET 1 answers

Determine which response is true or false regarding patient rights and responsibility

YES	NO	RESPONSE
X		11. Receive respect and efficient care
	X	12. No need to know their diagnosis
	X	13. Receive informed consent after the treatment
	X	14. Not allowed to refuse treatment
X		15. Maintain confidentiality
X		16. Examine their bill for charges incurred
X		17. Can decide if wants to follow physician's instruction
X		18. Provide past medical history
	X	19. Determine if services should be paid
X		20. Provided privacy

Using the responses provided above, list which is a patient right and which is a patient responsibility.

11. __RIGHT___
12. _____
13. _____
14. _____
15. ___RIGHT_____
16. ___RIGHT_____
17. __RESPONSIBILITY_____
18. __RESPONSIBILTY_____
19. _____
20. __RIGHT_____

3. Does the unwritten agreement between a patient and the doctor end completely after the patient had been rendered care and the bill paid? Explain your response. Discharge of the patient usually ceases the relationship between the patient and the doctor. There are situations in which the doctor may continue the relationship, such as surgical patients may need follow-up assessments post discharge.
4. Can the physician cease care if the patient is non-compliant with the ordered regime? Explain your response. No. The physician must document the patient's response. The physician can tell the patient to seek another doctor and give a timeline on when current treatment will cease.

PEDIATRICS 1 answers

1. Explain the relationship between premature infants and lack of the physical development of the various body systems. Preterm or premature infants often have difficulty breathing and feeding as their organs are under developed. They also have the risk of a brain hemorrhage.

2. List a physical issue that may present in a premature male infant. Premature male infants may be born with hypospadias or scrotal abnormalities

3. Explain the reflex problems that occur when attempting to feed a premature infant. Preterm infants have difficulty feeding as they may present with impairment of the lips and jaws, as well as trouble swallowing. Preterm infants may not have fully developed digestive systems.

4. Briefly explain why premature infants have respiratory issues. Include in your response how surfactant plays a role in this issue. Preterm infants do not have fully developed lungs which can result in the babies ability to make surfactant. Surfactant assists the lungs to smoothly inflate and collapse. When there is too little surfactant, the lungs collapse and makes it very difficult for the baby to reinflate the lungs.

5. Explain why heat loss is a major concern in the premature infant. Include in your response, two interventions that the nurse may use to help prevent heat loss. Moving air across the infants skin causes convective heat loss. Lying the infant on a cold table results in conduction heat loss. Heat also evaporates from the infants wet skin. The nurse can place a hat on the infants head, use warm water to clean the infant, keep the infant wrapped in a blanket, and place under heating lamps.

6. What type of issues may present in the infant of diabetic mother. The infant may have low blood sugar at birth.

7. List two factors that may occur to the placenta during pregnancy and how it would influence the growth or survival of the fetus. Maternal hypertension can result in less blood reaching the placenta. Placental abruption is when the placenta partly or completely strip away from the uterus. If early in the pregnancy, the pregnancy would terminate. If late in the pregnancy, the baby would be emergently delivered.

8. Define brown fat and its purpose. Brown fat is fat stored until the body needs help maintaining the temperature. The brown fat is then broken down to create heat and raise the body temperature.

9. Define respiratory distress syndrome and its etiology. Respiratory distress syndrome is when the preterm infant is born with insufficient amounts of surfactant resulting in difficulty breathing.

Match the following.

	Definition	Correct response
1. Moro reflex	When infant cheek touched, the infant searches for a nipple in attempt to feed	3.
2. Palmer reflex	When lateral foot stroked, the big toe moves upward and the toes fan outward	4.
3. Rooting reflex	Infant grasps finger when placed in the hand	2.
4. Babinski reflex	Infant placed supine & downward extends then abducts extremities	1.

PEDIATRICS 2 answers

Match the age with the developmental milestone

1. Two months old	a. Rolls over
2. Four months old	b. Runs
3. Six months old	c. Holds cup
4. Nine months old	d. undresses self
5. Twelve months old	e. crawls
6. Eighteen months old	f. sits
7. Two years old	g. laughs
8. Three years old	h. Holds head up

2. __H_ 2. __A__ 3. __C____ 4. __E__ 5. __F___ 6. _D____ 7. __G__ 8. __B___

A. List two types of infant injuries that are commonly seen. Include how they could be prevented in your response. Fractures from falls. Place in crib with rails up. Ensure gaits at stairs. Poisoning from getting into cleaning agents under sinks or bathrooms.

B. What is separation anxiety? An exaggerated response from separated from a parent or guardian.

C. List two types of toddler injuries that are commonly seen. Include how they could be prevented in your response. Burns and drowning. Keep gaits up to prevent toddler from entering areas with stoves or grills. Safety gait on entrance to pools. Never leave a toddler in a tub alone.

D. What is parallel play? Two children play separately in the same area.

PEDIATRICS 3 answers

Complete the following with the timeline of when the vaccines should be administered.

Hepatitis A	12 months
Hepatitis B	18 months
Rotavirus	2 months
DTAP	2 months
Polio	2 months
Varicella	12 months
MMR	12 months
Influenza	6 months

Define the following.

1. Celiac's disease: An immune reaction to eating gluten.

2. Short bowel syndrome: The malabsorption of food in the small intestine

3. Cleft palate: A birth defect of the roof of the mouth.

4. Cleft lip: A birth defect of the lips

5. Spina bifida: A birth defect in which the spinal cord does not develop properly

6. What physical findings would you expect to observe in an infant with increased intracranial pressure? Bulging fontanels and the infant would be extremely irritable.

7. What is shaken baby syndrome? Include in your response signs you would observe if this occurred. An injury to the baby's brain as a result of forceful shaking of the baby. Symptoms may be drowsiness, vomiting, irritability, and difficulty breathing.

8. What is a febrile seizure? A seizure that occurs due to high fevers.

RESPIRATORY 1 answers

1. Define the following. Explain when it may be ordered.

PFT	Pulmonary function test are to assess how well the lungs are working.
ABG	Arterial blood gas is used to measure the levels of oxygen and carbon dioxide in the blood. This can determine the pH level.
Bronchoscopy	A procedure using a bronchoscope (tube that visualizes the are of the scope to assess the airways and diagnose lung issues
Thoracentesis	A thoracentesis is a procedure that is used to drain fluid that accumulates in the pleural space.
Pulse oximetry	A small device used to measure oxygen saturation
Nebulizer treatment	A medical machine that allows delivery of medication to the patient via a face mask to assist to improve breathing

2. Why must an Allen's test be completed before an ABG is performed?
To ensure adequate blood to the hand prior to drawing the arterial blood gas and applying pressure to the chosen artery.

3. In what position should the nurse place the patient when a thoracentesis will be performed?

> The patient should be sitting, with arms placed on the over-the-bed table for support. This allows better access to insert the needle between the ribs. If the patient is unable to sit, the patient can be placed in a side-lying position.

4. List reasons that may result in in inaccurate pulse oximetry readings.

> Cool or cold fingers. Shivering. Excessive movement. Poor circulation (Raynaud's disease or Berger's disease. Irregular heart rate. Probe placement inappropriate. Nail polish. Excessive light. Broken device.

5. What is the purpose of a chest tube?

> A chest tube is inserted to remove air or fluid (purulent drainage, blood, effusions), in the intrathoracic space.

6. When should a chest tube be removed?

> The chest tube should be removed when the amount of drainage has been low or has ceased or there is no air being removed from the chest.

RESPIRATORY 2 answers

1. A chest tube drainage system has three chambers. Name and list the purpose of each chamber.

The suction chamber	The chamber provides suction to assist in lung expansion. The doctor orders the amount of suction desired.
The water seal chamber	This chamber keeps the suction at a regulated pressure with a one-way valve that only allows air to exit the patient
The collection chamber	This chamber collects fluid that has been drained from the chest.

2. Explain how the nurse can confirm there is an air leak in the chest tube system.

> The chest tube drainage system often contains a meter that can determine an air leak. Chest tube drainage systems that do not have this meter, will require chest X-rays to determine worsening pneumothorax.

3. How can the nurse assess the cause of an air leak?

> If the water seal chamber no longer has bubbles, the air leak can be determined to be from the chest tube insertion site or within the patient's chest.

4. What is a sucking chest wound and what might be its cause?

> A sucking chest wound is an injury resulting in a hole in the chest. It can be caused by trauma such as a stabbing or gunshot wound (GSW).

5. What action should the nurse take if a chest tube is accidently disconnected?

> If the chest tube has been completely removed from the patient, pressure should be applied to the chest tube insertion site and a gauze pressure dressing applied to the site. IF the tubing of the chest tube is disconnected from the drainage system, new tubing should attached to the drainage system and reattached to the patient's chest tube.

6. What does it mean if the fluid in the water seal chamber rises and falls when the patient is breathing normally? Should the doctor be notified?

> This is normal. It is called tidaling. Tidaling confirms a patent chest tube.

RESPIRATORY 3 answers

1. Listed are six non-invasive oxygen delivery devices. List how much oxygen each deliver.

Nasal cannula	2 – 6 L/min. 24 - 40 % oxygen delivery
Simple mask	6 – 10 L/Min. 35 - 55 % oxygen delivery
Venturi mask	4 – 12 L/Min. 24 – 60 % measured oxygen flow
Face tent	15 L/Min. 28 -100 % oxygen delivery
Non-rebreather	10 – 15 L/Min. 85 - 90% oxygen via a face mask with a reservoir bag
BIPAP	Settings per physicians order. 35 – 100% FIO2

2. What is oxygen toxicity and how does it occur?

> Oxygen toxicity is damage that occurs to the lungs due to excessive oxygen consumption. The patient may be using more oxygen than required.

3. What is an endotracheal tube?

> An endotracheal tube is a tube inserted into the respiratory system (through the vocal cords) into the trachea. This tube is attached to a ventilator.

4. Define the difference between the following.

BIPAP	CPAP	Mechanical ventilation
The BIPAP uses different pressures for inspiration and expiration	The CPAP provides a constant pressure throughout the respiratory cycle.	The ventilator controls the entire breathing process of the patient.

Ex: inspiration 12 (I-12) Expiration 8 (E- 8)	Ex: 10 cmH20	Ex: RR 12, TV 500 FIO2 60% PEEP 5

5. Your patient's ventilator alarm keeps alarming because your patient has a leak in the endotracheal tubes balloon. Can you turn off the ventilator alarm to allow your patient to get some sleep? Explain your answer.

No. If the alarm is off and the breathing tube becomes occluded or is accidently removed, there will no warning to notify the nurse or staff. The nurse would not recognize the patient needed assistance.

RESPIRATORY 4 answers

1. Define the following.

Word	Define
Cyanosis	Inadequate oxygenation. Usually seen in nail beds as a blue color
Hypoxemia	Low concentrations of oxygen within the blood
Hypoventilation	Very low respiratory rate. May include shallow respirations
PEEP	Positive end-expiratory pressure. It is the pressure in the lungs at the end of expiration that keeps the alveoli open
Acidosis	The body has too much acidity.
Alkalosis	The body has too much base.
VAP	Ventilator-associated pneumonia. Pneumonia is diagnosed 48 hours or more after the patient is intubated and placed on a ventilator
Barotrauma	Excessive pressure resulting in tissue damage. The lungs may be overstretched. This condition can occur in body cavities such as the sinus from fluid build up

Atelectasis	The lung is unable to expand completely.
Pleural effusions	Abnormal fluid accumulation in the pleural space.
ARDS	Acute respiratory distress syndrome. A condition of fluid build up within the lungs.
Wheezes	Adventitious lungs sounds that produce a high-pitched sound
Crackles	Adventitious lung sounds usually auscultated during inspiration
Rales	Rattling sounds auscultated during inspiration.
Rhonchi	Coarse, low pitched wheezy breath sounds auscultated in the lungs.

2. What is a stridor? A stridor is a partial obstruction in the airflow during inspiration. Often heard in the patient status post (S/P) extubation.

RESPIRATORY 5 answers

1. Match the following ventilator settings to their definition

Ventilator setting	definition
Assist control ventilation	Preset rate and tidal volume that will be given. Patient may breathe spontaneously in between set rate.
Synchronized intermittent mandatory ventilation	The ventilator adds pressure at the end of each breath to keep the alveoli open to promote gas exchange
Pressure support ventilation	Preset rate and tidal volume. Patient may initiate the breath but ventilator delivers the tidal volume for each breath taken. Client may breathe above set rate
Positive end expiratory pressure	Patient initiates rate and tidal volume but assistance is given by the ventilator during inspirations

2. Explain the difference between rhinitis and a common cold.

Rhinitis.	Common cold

| Rhinitis is an allergic reaction to an allergen. | A virus that results in an illness that affects the nose and throat. May include, stuffy nose, runny nose, cough, sinus drainage, hoarse throat. |

3. What is the relationship between pneumonia and influenzas? Influenza is an illness that can cause aches, hyperthermia, vomiting. Pneumonia can be a complication of influenza. Pneumonia can also have other causes. Aspiration. Bacterial. Ventilator associated pneumonia.

4. What is the difference between an epidemic and a pandemic?

Epidemic	pandemic
An epidemic is the spread of a disease in a select population	A pandemic is the spread of a disease that spreads through a very large population or worldwide.

RESPIRATORY 6 answers

1. In a patient diagnosed with pneumonia, what findings would you expect to see in the following?

WBC	Elevated due to infection
ABG	Respiratory acidosis. Low oxygen. High CO2
SPUTUM SPECIMEN	Positive for bacteria
BLOOD CULTURES	Positive for bacteria

2. A Patient with a history of asthma begins to wheeze. Should you be concerned? Explain your response. Wheezing indicates narrowing of the airway and may result in bronchoconstriction. This can cause respiratory compromise.

3. List the four categories of asthma.

Category 1	Mild and intermittent symptoms occur two or less times weekly
Category 2	Mild persistent symptoms that occur once daily or 2 + times weekly
Category 3	Moderate persistent symptoms occur daily and increased risk to progress to severe
Category 4	Severe persistent symptoms occur throughout the entire day. Difficulty to do activities of daily living.

4. List four triggers of asthma.

Animal dander
mold
Dust mites
pollen

5. What is status asthmaticus?

Acute bout of asthma that fails to respond to therapy. This is a medical emergency.

6. You notice your patient has been having labored breathing is showing signs of sternal retraction. What does sternal retractions indicate?

This is an indication that the patient is using accessory muscles to breath. It is a sign of respiratory distress.

RESPIRATORY 7 answers

1. Define the following. List a known cause of each.

Disease	Definition	cause
COPD	Chronic inflammatory disease of the lung	Inhaled pollutants such as smoking, job related dust (coal), air pollution.
Emphysema	Alveoli of the lungs are damaged resulting in difficulty exhaling	Smoking, pollutants such as job related dust (coal).
Bronchitis	Inflammation of the upper airway	Infection.

2. Which respiratory disease may present with a barrel chest?
   The emphysema patient can be seen with a barrel chest.
   3. What is incentive spirometry and what is its use in a patient with a respiratory disease?
      An incentive spirometry is a device that assists to open up the alveoli of the lungs. This device assist to improve ventilation.

4. List a non-respiratory response of a bronchodilator medication. Headache, shakiness, or tachycardia.

5. When the nurse instructs the patient to "smell the flowers (slowly inhale) and blow out the candles (slowly exhale)," this practice is to teach to the patient to do what?
The nose warms air as well as filters out toxins. This technique also helps the patient to take deep breaths.

6. What is T.B.?
T.B. abbreviated for tuberculosis is a highly contagious infection usually affecting the lungs.

7. What pathogen can be seen in a patient diagnosed with T.B.? mycobacterium tuberculosis.

8. What type of isolation should a patient with active T.B. be placed? Airborne isolation precautions should be taken.

9. Does T.B. only affect the lungs? Explain your response. No. T.B. can affect other organs of the body.

RESPIRATORY 8 answers

1. What is another name for an intradermal test?

Allergy testing. For T.B. it is the Mantoux test.

2. Define the following different ways to test for T.B.

Mantoux tests	An intradermal injection of 0.1 ml of tuberculin)PPD) to test for exposure to T.B.
Quantiferon test	This is considered the gold standard to test for T.B. A laboratory blood test
AFB test	Acid-fast bacteria culture specimen (sputum) used to test for T.B.

3. What type of mask should a nurse wear when caring for a patient with active TB?
An N95 test fitted respiratory mask.

4. When a Mantoux test is administered, when should the results be read? For a health care professional, a Mantoux test should be administered prior to employment and annually thereafter. The Mantoux test should be read 48 – 72 hours after administration of the test.

5. Determine the results of the following Mantoux readings.

Results	Population	Positive or negative
"0" mm	Nursing assistant	negative
Less than "5" mm	A patient with no risk factors	negative
Greater than "5"mm	A HIV positive patient	positive
Greater than "10" mm	A patient with no risk factors	positive
Greater than "10"mm	A patient who uses DOA	Positive
Greater than "15"mm	A patient with no risk factors	positive. May react to previous vaccine
Greater than "15"mm	A patient with allergies	Positive

6. A patient has a history of T.B. The patient has been taking the prescribed medication for 11 months. Does this patient require isolation? Explain your response. Yes. The patient should be place in isolation until the threat of active T.B. is ruled out.

RESPIRATORY 9 answers

1. Define the following, when they might occur, and the cause.

Pulmonary emboli	Blood clot in the lung blocks a pulmonary artery. A clot forms in the lower body (DVT) and travels to the lung
Pleurisy	An inflammation in the parietal or visceral layers of the lung. Can be caused by an infection.
Pleural friction rub	The sound of two pleural tissue rub together creating a rubbing sound that is heard during inspiration and expiration

2. What is an IVC filter?
An IVC filter is an inferior vena cava filter that is placed in the inferior vena cava to stop blood clots from entering the lung.
3. Define the following and how they relate to a PE.

Test/procedure/symptom	Define	How relates to a PE
Embolectomy	The surgical removal of a blood clot	An embolectomy removes a clot that is blocking perfusion and is too large to treat with medication
VQ scan	A ventilation perfusion scan that assesses the air flow and the blood flow through the lungs	This test is used to diagnose pulmonary emboli in the lungs
PET scan	A positron emission tomography is an imaging test that assesses organs & blood flow	A PET scan can show the location of an emboli, it is not the best choice. A pulmonary angiography is best.
Petechiae	Bleeding under the skin that are seen as pin point spots on the skin	Petechiae may appear if due to capillary ruptures.

4. What interventions can be done for the patient with a PE? (Remember medications). The intervention depends on the severity of the clot. A thrombectomy, embolectomy, and anticoagulants. Usually a continuous heparin infusion is uses unless an allergy is noted. Argatroban can be used.

RESPIRATORY 10 answers

1. What is the difference between a pneumothorax (PTX) and a hemothorax?

   A pneumothorax occurs when air enters the pleural space causing the lung to collapse (may be partial or a full collapse). This can occur from a bleb. A hemothorax is when blood enters into the pleural space causing the lung to collapse. This can occur from a trauma (stab wound or gunshot wound).

2. Define the following and how it relates to a PTX.

	Define	How it relates to a PTX
Bleb	A gas filled cyst-like tissue often attached to the lung pleura.	When a bleb ruptures, it can cause a spontaneous pneumothorax.
Flail chest	When multiple ribs are detached from the rib cage, the chest appears to have	A pneumothorax is often a complication of a flail chest. The broken ribs may puncture

		paradoxical movements.	the lung.
Tracheal deviation		The trachea moves to one side as a result of abnormal pressure in the chest	A tension pneumothorax can cause increased pressure in the chest, causing tracheal deviation

3. List symptoms of respiratory distress.

Tachypnea
Shallow respirations
Tachycardia
Cyanosis of the nail beds
Short of breath
Nasal flaring
Sternal retraction
Use of respiratory accessory muscles
Difficulty in breathing

4. When a tracheal deviation occurs, in which direction does it deviate?
   The trachea will deviate toward the lung that has collapsed.
5. What is the difference between an internal and external PTX? An internal PTX is when the air from the lungs enters the pleural cavity. An external PTX is when air enters the pleural space from outside the body.
6. What is a sucking chest wound? A sucking chest wound is an open pneumothorax. Air from the atmosphere enters the pleural space resulting in lung collapse.

RESPIRATORY 11 answers

1. Explain the pathophysiology of how asthma occurs.

After exposure to an allergen, the airways become irritated. The airways swell, create mucus which often causes more narrowing of the airway. The muscles tighten around the airway making it more difficult to breath. Asthma is a chronic airway disorder that can result in bronchial hyperresponsiveness, obstruction of the airway, and inflammation.

2. Explain why the doctor would order a nebulizer treatment for an asthmatic patient. What does a nebulizer treatment do?

A nebulizer treatment is administered via a machine that converts medication to a mist that allows the medication easier entry into the lungs. Often these nebulizer treatments aid to relax the muscles and loosens up mucus resulting in better airway flow.

3. List three initial interventions that may be used on an asthmatic patient. Explain your rationale for each intervention.

> 1. Assess oxygenation status. Auscultate lungs. Apply pulse oximetry. The nurse must first assess before planning any intervention.
> 2. Position the head of bed at high Fowlers. In the high Fowler's position, gravity assists to move the diaphragm downward aiding in lung expansion.
> 3. Administer medication. The medication can aid to open up the airways.

4. Your asthmatic patient states he has been using his inhalers as ordered. How can you be certain the patient is using his inhalers correctly? Explain your response.

> Ask the patient to demonstrate how he uses the inhaler. This way you can document if the patient is using the inhaler correctly or if the patient needs further patient education.

5. Explain how you would teach your patient how to use an inhaler. How can you be certain your patient understands the instructions correctly? Explain your response.

> Ensure the inhaler is the correct inhaler and not expired. Remove the cap. Some respiratory therapist will gently shake the inhaler. The patient should be instructed to breath out slowly and completely. Place the inhaler to the mouth and administer the dose as the patient inhales quickly and deeply. Remove the inhaler and instruct the patient to exhale slowly. Ask your patient to return demonstration of the steps he was just instructed to perform.

RESPIRATORY 12 answers

1. Where would you auscultate and find the following?

Sounds	Location
Bronchial lung sounds	On lateral sides of the trachea, above the clavicles
Bronchovesicular lung sounds	Between the 1st and 2nd intercostal space, lateral to the sternum. Posteriorly between the scapula.
Vesicular lung sounds	Below the 2nd rib, throughout the remaining lung fields to the lung bases.

2. What is adventitious breath sounds and what would be their cause(s)? Wheezes and crackles that occur in conditions such as asthma or bronchitis.
3. List 4 different pulmonary diseases and what lung sounds you would hear with each.

    Rhonchi: COPD

    Wheezes: Asthma. COPD

    Crackles: Congestive heart failure, COPD, or pneumonia

    Stridor: Asthma

4. Describe techniques for auscultating lung sounds. Using the diaphragm of the stethoscope, place the diaphragm on the skin (not on the gown) and in a systematic way, auscultate the anterior, lateral and posterior chest area. Have the patient take deep breaths (inspiratory and expiratory) through the mouth.
5. Identify why it is important to auscultate the lungs prior and after performing nasotracheal suctioning. To asses if the suctioning cleared secretions and improved breath sounds.
6. If your patient had a lobectomy, would it be necessary to auscultate for lung sounds over the "missing" lung site? Explain your response. Yes. Lung sounds will be diminished.
7. Your patient's son insists his mother (your patient) do abdominal breathing only while awake. What is abdominal breathing? Abdominal breathing or belly breathing is a technique that strengthens the diaphragm which in turn assists to fill the lungs.
8. How would you respond to the patient's son? If the patient agrees, the patient will be encouraged to use diaphragmatic breathing techniques.
9. Your patient has Raynaud's disease and the pulse oximetry placed on her finger shows a pulse oximetry level of 58%. What would be your next actions to ensure adequate oxygenation. Some pulse oximetry can be placed on the earlobes. If unable to use the pulse oximetry, notify the doctor. If the patient requires, an arterial blood gas can be ordered.

SPINAL 1 answers

1. Explain why the loss of functional ability is determined by the level of injury to the spinal cord.

    The higher the injury of the spine, the greater area that is affected which may result in paralysis.

2. Why is immobilization important when a spinal injury occurs? Immobilization is important to prevent damage to the spinal cord. Broken bones can severe nerves. Misalignment may cause complications. Immobilization is best to prevent further injury.
3. Define autonomic dysreflexia? Autonomic dysreflexia is an abnormal reaction of the autonomic

    nervous system. This can occur from stimulation (autonomic = involuntary)

4. What is spinal shock? Spinal shock is the impairment below the level of injury to the spine. This

    can result in paralysis, loss of bowel/bladder control, and loss of reflexes.

5. At what level of injury would the patient's ability to breath independently be compromised? Cervical spinal injuries that occur at level C1, C2, or C3 will require mechanical ventilation as they are unable to breath independently.

6. List the potential health concerns a male patient may have if diagnosed with paralysis below the waist. Besides loss of bowel and bladder, the patient may also have erectile dysfunction.

7. What does it mean if the patient is quadriplegic? Quadriplegic is the name for paralysis from the neck down. This includes paralysis of the extremities.

8. What does it mean if the patient is paraplegic? Paraplegic is the name for paralysis of the lower half of the body.

9. If the doctor tells the patient his severity of injury is complete, what does it mean? Complete means there is no muscle control, sensation or feeling or function below the injury.

10. If the doctor tells the patient his severity of injury is incomplete, what does it mean? There is some degree of movement, or sensation/feeling below the injury.

STATE BOARD REVIEW PRACTICE 1 answers

Using the tables below, choose the most appropriate response.

Your Parkinson's patient's wife asks you how is Parkinson diagnosed. You explain ____(2)_____.

Table A
1. With a computed tomography (CT) scan
2. By presenting symptoms, family observations, and past medical history
3. Magnetic resonance imaging (MRI) scan

The patient's wife then asks, "How long will it take to cure my husband of this Parkinsons?" You reply _____(3)_____.

Table B
1. With exercise, diet and medication, it may resolve within four months
2. Every patient responds differently to treatment. It cannot be predicted
3. Symptoms can be managed with medication. Parkinsons disease is a progressive disease with no cure

The patient's wife asks, "Is there anything I should be made aware of when caring for my husband?"

You reply _____(1)_____.

Table C
1. He may have swallowing issues as the disease progresses. He may choke.
2. People may point and stare when his tremors worsen.
3. There are no concerns to worry about.

STATE BOARD REVIEW PRACTICE 2 answers

Using the tables below, choose the most appropriate response.

Your patient asks you what is Alzheimer's disease. You explain ____(1)_____.

Table A
1. A progressive neurodegenerative disease
2. A disease that only affects the elderly who are older than 70 years and sickly
3. A communicable disease that can be spread by respiratory droplets

The patient then asks, "What are the risk factors?" You reply _____(3)_____.

Table B
1. Daily exercise, low fat diet, and low carbohydrate intake
2. Low cholesterol, hypoglycemia, and low blood pressure
3. Hypertension, diabetes, obesity, smoking, and hyperlipidemia

The patient asks, "Are there any signs?"

You reply _____(1)_____.

Table C
1. Forgetfulness, memory loss, and difficulty with words
2. Able to flawlessly recall long-term memory and short-term memory information
3. Begins to take a higher interest in completing routine tasks

STATE BOARD REVIEW PRACTICE 3 answers

Using the tables below, choose the most appropriate response.

Your patient asks you what is Lou Gerig's disease. You explain ___2_____.

Table A
1. A disease known as "dropsy". Labeled after a cherry picker.
2. A disease that causes loss of motor neurons. Labeled after a baseball player.
3. A disease resulting in repetitive speech. Labeled after a radio host.

The patient then asks, "Are there early signs?" You reply _____1_____.

Table B

1. Slurred speech, weakness, and tripping.
2. "Second sight" and hyper-reflexive grasps.
3. Manic episodes with surges of nervous energy.

The patient asks, "Is there a cure?"

You reply _____2_____.

Table C
1. With an implanted deep-brain stimulator.
2. Medications that increase the production of Glutamate.
3. Non-curable degenerative neuromuscular disease

STATE BOARD REVIEW PRACTICE 4 answers

Using the tables below, choose the most appropriate response.

Your patient asks you can he recover from a brain tumor. You explain ____1_____.

Table A
1. The prognosis would depend on the type of tissue, location, and intervention.
2. Absolutely. Medicine has achieved a lot of success with laser surgeries.
3. Yes. Brain tumors are slow growing and can be reduced with radiation therapy.

The patient then asks, "What are the signs of a brain tumor?" You reply _____2_____.

Table B

356

1. Rigid stance with an inability to bend at the waist.
2. Headaches that worsen at night.
3. Inability to tolerate spicy odors

The patient asks, "how do you test for a brain tumor?"

You reply _____1_____.

Table C
1. An extensive neurological examination and past medical history.
2. By obtaining a mammogram with contrast
3. By using a tuning fork. Striking the tuning fork and touching the center lower jaw

TEST YOUR KNOWLEDGE 1 answers

Define the following:

1. Sediment: matter that is present in a liquid

2. Donning: putting on

3. Ashen: gray color

4. Dusky: dark colored

5. Pallor: loss of color

6. Ruberous: redness

7. Cyanotic: bluish color

8. Edema: swelling of body tissue

9. Dehiscence: separation of a wound

10. Hyperthermia: body temperature above normal

Define the following abbreviations:

11. PVD: peripheral vascular disease

12. CHF: congestive heart failure

13. MI: myocardial infarction

14. CVA: cerebral vascular accident

15. MVC: motor vehicle crash

16. JVD: jugular vein distention

17. SC: subcutaneous

18. IM: intramuscular

TEST YOUR KNOWLEDGE 2 answers

1. Explain the difference between an AV graft and an AV fistula. An AV graft connects the artery to a vein via a tube and graft. Whereas, an AV fistula connects the artery and vein together directly.

2. If a patient's A1C is greater than 7, would this confirm the patient was compliant with her diabetic regime? Explain your response. If the patient is taking an antidiabetic medication the A1C should be below 7. This may mean the patient is non-compliant or the patient's condition is worsening.

3. Explain how each of the following topics are complications of diabetes.

    d. Macular degeneration: this condition affects the macula of the eye and is a complication of diabetes.

    e. Neuropathy: nerve damage that is caused by high levels of glucose in the blood from diabetes.

    f. Hair loss: Loss of hair due to poor circulation from high glucose levels

4. List the interventions for each of the following basic care and comfort issues.

    e. Hygiene: the patient may not be able to care for themselves. Cleansing the skin, washing the hair, shaving, the patient provides basic care and comfort.

    f. Progressive mobility: Patients with health issues (CVA) that can not move themselves, will require progressive mobility (assist to chair, proper body alignment) or Passive-range-of motion to make the patient feel comfortable and provide care.

    g. Nutrition: Meals can aid in making the patient feel well cared for.

    h. Pain control: A patient who is experiencing pain, can not sleep well, feel comfortable sitting or interacting. Providing pain management can provide care and comfort.

5. Why is it important to have an advanced directive? This can provide a guide for the health care team to honor the patient's wishes and eliminate the burden on their family members.

6. What is a bruit and thrill? A bruit is the sound blood makes when moving through the AV graft or AV fistula. The thrill can be palpated on the AV graft or AV fistula.

7. What sign is positive when tested for the patient with a diagnosis of meningitis? The Brudzinski's sign is positive in meningitis. When the neck is flexed the patient's hip and knees flex.

8. What is myelopathy? Compression to the spinal cord due to a herniated disc, or injury.

9. Why is it important to know the chain of command? It ensure accountability at each level.

10. What equipment should every nurse have readily available daily? A pen, a pen light, a pair of scissors (trauma scissors preferred), a notebook, and a watch with a second hand.

TEST YOUR KNOWLEDGE 3 answers

1. Define encephalitis and potential causes. Encephalitis is inflammation of the brain. This inflammation may be caused by bacterial or viral infections.

2. List three clinical symptoms that may present in the patient with encephalitis. Include one laboratory result in your response. Headache, hyperthermia, photophobia. Laboratory test can include spinal fluid analysis (lumbar puncture), and ammonia levels.

3. What is Reyes syndrome and what population of patients is it most commonly seen? A condition that causes swelling in the brain status post (S/P) infection. The age group mostly affected are children and teens.

4. Define Sepsis: A response to an infection that result in organ failure and death if not diagnosed early.

5. Are there early signs of sepsis that can be monitored for to assist to prevent it from becoming severe? Explain your response. Yes. Hyperthermia. shivering, confusion, tachycardia, low urine output. These are early signs of sepsis.

6. What does it mean to pan culture the patient? To send multiple specimens. Blood cultures, urine cultures, and sputum cultures.

7. What is a seizure? Include two causes of seizures. Trauma to the head can result in a seizure. Hyperthermia can result in a febrile seizure.

8. What is status epilepticus? A seizure with a duration of 5 minutes or greater or the occurrence of seizure activity without recovery between them.

9. What is autism? Include how it is diagnosed in your response. A neurological developmental disorder that causes social interaction issues, communication issues, as well as behavioral issues. A specialist will diagnose autism from observed behaviors.

10. What is the difference between cardiomegaly and cardiomyopathy? Cardiomegaly is the enlargement of the heart as a result of damage to the heart muscle. Cardiomyopathy is the enlargement of the heart which grows weaker. Also known as dilated heart.

11. What is meningitis? Inflammation of the meninges of the brain.

12. What is Kerning's sign? A test to determine meningeal irritation.

13. Explain the relationship between epilepsy and seizures. Epilepsy is abnormal electrical brain activity resulting in 2 or more seizures within a 24 hour period. Seizures can occur for other reasons. Such as a febrile seizure or trauma to the head.

14. What is Cerebral palsy? Include potential causes in your response. Cerebral palsy is damage to the brain that occurs more often prior to birth.

15. Define the following:
    a. Ataxia: poor muscle control
    b. Nystagmus: Repetitive, uncontrolled movement of the eye.
    c. Decerebrate: Posturing resulting in the extremities extended and rigid.
    d. Decorticate: posturing resulting in flexion of the arms while extension of the lower extremities.

URINARY SYSTEM 1 answers

Match the following

1. _C_   2. _F_   3. _G_   4. _E_   5. _D_   6. _H_   7. _B_   8. _A_

Fill in the blank

1. Dark urine indicates dehydration.
2. Pale urine indicates adequate hydration.

1. Polyuria	a. The retention of waste and metabolites
2. Oliguria	b. Leukocytes in the urine
3. Proteinuria	c. Elimination of large amounts of urine
4. Glucosuria	d. Sign of incomplete fat metabolism
5. Ketonuria	e. Exceeds blood glucose reabsorption capability
6. Hematuria	f. Urine output of 400 ml or less daily
7. Pyuria	g. Protein in the urine
8. Azotemia	h. Red blood cells in the urine

3. Rust colored urine indicates the presence of blood which can be due to kidney or liver disease.
4. The urine will have a fruity odor if glucose is present.
5. Specific gravity is normally 1.005 to 1.030.

List the three phases of acute renal failure (now called acute renal injury).

a. pre-renal (compromised renal perfusion)

b. renal (kidney function grossly reduced or fail to work)

c. post-renal (obstruction below kidneys (in the urinary tract) result in waste build up.

List three pre-renal failure causes.

a. hypovolemia (kidneys are sensitive to low fluid intake resulting in impaired renal clearance)

b. hypotension (results in low flow and low filtration resulting in renal failure)

c. medications (NSAIDS and some antibiotics can cause kidney injury)

URINARY SYSTEM 2 answers

1. List three causes of chronic renal failure.
   a. diabetes
   b. high blood pressure
   c. heart disease

2. Explain why acidosis occurs when the kidneys fail. The kidneys which produce bicarbonate through the process of ammoniagenesis, is unable to perform this process when the glomerular filtration rate is low. Without bicarbonate, the kidneys cannot neutralize the acids produced by the body resulting in metabolic acidosis.

3. Explain why anemia is prevalent in chronic renal failure. When the kidneys fail, they cannot make erythropoietin. Erythropoietin is a hormone secreted by the kidneys that stimulates bone marrow to produce red blood cells. Without adequate erythropoietin, the patient becomes anemic.

4. Explain what is erythropoietin and its role in renal failure? Erythropoietin is a hormone secreted by the kidneys. With lower or no erythropoietin, the body does not have enough red blood cells. This leads to anemia.

5. Define osteomalacia and explain its relationship to renal failure. Osteomalacia is soft or weakened bones. Patients in renal failure are unable to absorb phosphates which result in osteomalacia.

6. What is uremic frost? Patients in renal failure have a build up of waste products in the blood due to the kidneys inability to filter effectively. White urea crystals deposit onto the skin giving the impression of frost. It is itchy (mostly at night).

7. List a nursing intervention for a patient in renal failure with uremic frost. Patient teaching. A renal diet, what foods, beverages, and medications (NSAIDS) to avoid. Monitor blood pressure. Be active (exercise).

8. Why must a patient in renal failure have to be concerned about their cardiac status. Explain your response. Renal failure increases the risk of heart disease due to the added pressure (high blood pressure). The body attempts to help the kidneys by producing hormones to elevate the blood pressure in efforts to increase blood flow to the kidneys. This elevated systemic pressure that the heart must pump against. This can cause the heart to weaken from the additional workload and pressure.

9. Your patient has been diagnosed with renal failure. The patient asks, "what is dialysis? The doctor said I will need to have it." Explain what is dialysis and how would you explain it to your patient. Dialysis is a procedure to remove excess fluid and waste from the blood. The blood is cycled from the patient to an artificial kidney that will filter out excess fluid and waste and then the blood is returned to the patient.

10. Explain why monitoring intake and output is important when caring for a patient in renal failure. Patient's in renal failure are educated to understand the body can no longer remove excessive fluids without the aid of dialysis. Daily weights and monitoring intake and output can assist to maintain a fluid balance.

URINARY SYSTEM 3 answers

Define the following:

1. Nephrostomy: A drain placed in the kidney that exits through an opening in the skin.

2. Nephrectomy: the surgical removal of a kidney

3. Nephrolithotomy: a procedure to remove stones from the kidney

4. Pyelolithotomy: a surgical procedure to remove kidney stones.

5. Ureterolithotomy: a surgical procedure to remove kidney stones

6. Extracorporeal lithotripsy: non-invasive procedure that uses shock waves to break down kidney stones.

7. Cystitis: inflammation of the bladder due to bacterial infection.

8. Urethritis: inflammation of the urethra due to infection.

9. Extropy of the bladder: the bladder develops outside the fetus

10. Ileal conduit: A surgical urinary diversion that drains urine through a stoma.

11. Ureterostomy: A surgical procedure that diverts the urine from the ureter to a stoma.

12. Dialysis: a procedure to remove fluid and waste products from the blood.

Answer the following questions

1. Why is intake and output important in the renal failure patient? To ensure fluid overload does not occur.
2. Why must the patient be taught about dietary changes? To assist to maintain a better healthy state. Low protein diets have been shown to reduce glomerular pressure. The body needs calcium to assist bone development. High potassium levels can cause electrophysiological dysfunctions.
3. Why are laboratory results needed more often in the renal patient? To ensure the body's homeostasis is balanced. The doctor may need to add erythropoietin or vitamin D.
4. Why is it anticipated that the renal patient will become anemic? The kidneys need erythropoietin (a hormone) to stimulate red blood cell production. Renal failure patients are anemic due to lack of erythropoietin.

URINARY 4 answers

1. List four processes or systems that allow the body to maintain a water balance. Renin-angiotensin hormonal system (stimulates thirst), osmolality (blood concentrations trigger thirst), blood pressure baroreceptors (decreased blood volume triggers the heart to increase rate), kidneys (renin-angiotensin system) stimulates production of angiotensin II, releases aldosterone which in turn reabsorbs sodium in the distal tubules.

2. Osmoreceptors in which organ is responsible to stimulate thirst and antidiuretic hormone (ADH) from the posterior pituitary? The osmoreceptors in the hypothalamus signal the release of ADH from the posterior pituitary.

3. Which section of the kidneys does ADH act upon? ADH directs the epithelial cells (they line the collecting tubules in the kidneys) to increase water permeability.

4. Briefly explain what may be the body's main protection against dehydration and hyperosmolarity? The thirst mechanism kicks in when the body is dehydrated. When the body has less fluid, it becomes hyperosmolar (high levels of sodium and other substances). The osmoreceptors signals the hypothalamus which in turn triggers the thirst mechanism.

5. List three factors that may influence the secretion of ADH or the thirst mechanism. Osmolarity of the blood. The baroreceptors recognize a lower blood volume. The kidneys recognize low pressure.
6. Explain why the sedated post-surgical patient is at greater risk for a fluid deficit. The patient is unable to comprehend the thirst mechanism due to the sedative state. They are unable to eat or drink even if they were more alert due to post-surgical restrictions (NPO).

7. Explain why a dry mouth does not necessarily indicate a fluid deficit. The salivary glands may not produce enough saliva or the person is a mouth breather which dries out the mouth.

8. List two functions of the kidneys. To remove extra fluid from the body and to remove waste products.
9. List two health issues that may occur if the kidneys are not functioning properly. The body will become anemic and bone health will be compromised.

Determine which response below pertains to cortisol or aldosterone

RESPONSE	CORTISOL OR ALDOSTERONE
1. Responds to psychological stressors	cortisol
2. Responds to hypotension	aldosterone

3.	Anti-inflammatory effect	cortisol
4.	Enhances sodium retention	aldosterone
5.	Secreted during the circadian rhythm	cortisol

URINARY 5   answers

1. Why do burns cause trouble for the kidneys? Damaged muscles release myoglobin into the blood which can damage kidneys.
2. Does the geriatric patient have structural changes in the kidneys? Explain your response. Yes. The renal tissues change as the person ages resulting in decreased renal functioning.
3. Why are women more prone to urinary tract infections? Include one way to decrease or prevent these urinary tract infections. A woman's anatomy increases the risk of urinary tract infections. Bacteria (e-coli) from the anus can enter the urethra resulting in an infection. Ways to decrease or prevent urinary tract infections are to wipe from front to back, void after sex, and wear cotton underwear.
4. Define hypospadias and include potential health issues that may occur with this condition. Hypospadias is a birth condition where the meatus has not developed at the tip of the penis. Urethral strictures, abnormal chordee, curvature of the penis, and incomplete foreskin.
5. Define epispadias and include potential health issues that may occur with this condition. A birth defect in which the urethra does not fully form but exits from an abnormal location on the penis. May be surgically corrected but some patients may be rendered incontinent.

List why the following urine specimens would be ordered.

DEFINE	RESPONSE
1. Routine urine specimen	To assess the urine for disorders such as an infection, diabetes, ketones, or stones.
2. Sterile urine specimen	To ensure the specimen has not been contaminated with germs.
3. Clean catch or mid-stream urine specimen	To ensure the specimen has not been contaminated with germs.
4. Glucose, acetone, and protein in the urine specimen	Glucose maybe present if the patient is diabetic or pregnant. Acetone (ketones) may be present if the body breaks down fat cells. The presence of proteins in the urine may indicate a nephropathy.
5. 24-hour urine specimen	This test assists to diagnose renal problems. It measures the amount of creatinine clears through the kidneys

WORK SHEET – LABORATORY answers

Match the following

1. WBC – ELEVATED	
2. HgB - ELEVATED	
3. PLT - LOW	
4. POTASSIUM - ELEVATED	
5. SODIUM - ELEVATED	
6. WBC – LOW	
7. BUN – ELEVATED	
8. HgB – LOW	

A.	Neurological confusion
B.	Anemia
C.	Infection
D.	Potential for hemorrhage
E.	Potential for cardiac arrest
F.	Dehydration
G.	Cancer
H.	Renal failure

1. __C____. 2. __F_____. 3. _D_____. 4. _E_____. 5. ____A____. 6. __G_____.

7. __H_____. 8. ___B____.

Match the following

1.	Sodium
2.	Potassium
3.	Calcium
4.	Bicarb
5.	Magnesium

a. low level in a drug overdose
b. low levels seen in torsades
c. reduced by diuretics
d. Chvostek's sign seen with low levels
e. Low levels seen with SIADH

1. _E_____. 2. __C____. 3. _D_____. 4. _A_____. 5. ___B____.

WORKSHEET – BEST PRACTICES answers

1. What is the best position to place the patient for the nurse to assess for jugular vein distention (JVD)?

a. 90 degrees	b. Trendelenburg
c. 45 degrees	d. prone

   Answer: _____C_____

2. If having difficulty auscultating the heart. What position can the patient be placed to assist to better hear the heart sounds?

a. Sitting up, leaning on over the bed table	b. Lying flat, positioned on right side
c. Lying flat, positioned on left side	d. Lying flat, in supine position

   Answer: _____c._____

3. The patient is a quadriplegic. What areas would be prone to pressure ulcers? Mark all that apply

a. Scapula	b. vertebra	c. Anterior wrists
d. Elbows	e. Lateral shoulders	f. Medial ankles
g. Hips	h. Sacrum	i. Medial knees
j. Lateral knees	k. Heels	l. knuckles

   Answer(s): a, b, d, e, f, g, h, i, k.

4. The patient is lying flat in a supine position. The patient complains (C/O) difficulty in breathing. What is the FIRST action you could and should do?

   Answer: Elevate the head of the bed.

5. What is the first action the nurse should do before entering a patient's room?

   Answer: wash the hands or use hand gel.

WORKSHEET – INTAKE AND OUTPUT answers

The following are items of measure that the patient had during your shift. Calculate the intake and output and tally for your 8 hour shift.

Jello	6 ounces
Coffee	8 ounces
Bouillion	8 ounces
Urine output	240 ml
IV fluids	50 ml/Hr
IV piggyback	100 ml
Jello x 2	12 ounces
Tea	8 ounces
Water	500 ml
Urine output	650 ml
Emesis	100 ml

Total intake: __2260 ml__   Total output: ____990_____

Based on your calculations, is the patient euvolemic, overhydration, or underhydration?

Answer: ____overhydration_____

What is the total difference between the total intake and the total output?

Answer: _____1270 ml_____.

List what may be the cause of your difference in intake and output.

Patient may have been NPO for a day or two.
The patient may be in renal failure
The patient may have congestive heart failure
The patient may be dehydrated
Diarrhea
Fever
Excessive sweating

WORKSHEET - URINARY SYSTEM ANSWERS

Define the following urinary issues. Specify if it is an infection or a renal condition. compare the difference between acute and chronic, or listed issue, when applicable.

Condition or infection	Define	Compare	How is this issue diagnosed
1. Acute pyelonephritis: Sudden onset and may cause permanent damage to the kidneys	An inflammation of the kidneys caused by a bacterial infection	Chronic pyelonephritis Repetitive occurrences of kidney infections	A computed tomography (CT) scan, a magnetic resonance imaging (MRI), or an ultrasound can diagnose pyelonephritis
2. Acute glomerulonephritis: sudden onset due to infection resulting in inflammation of the glomeruli	Inflammation of the glomerulus	Chronic Glomerulonephritis: gradual onset of the inflammation of the glomeruli	Urine test Blood test (antinuclear antibody test) Renal ultrasound
3. Polycystic kidney: genetic mutation resulting in multiple fluid-filled cyst growing within the kidney		Renal calculi: kidney stones (crystals), or nephrolithiasis: form when too much of a substance is in the urine. Can be calcium, oxalate, or uric acid.	Renal ultrasound
4. Renal artery stenosis: narrowing of the renal arteries due to atherosclerosis	Narrowing	Urethral stricture: urethral lining becomes narrow to due injury (can be caused by surgical intervention)	Urethral stricture: cystoscopy Renal artery stenosis: ultrasound
5. Renal tuberculosis: lesions that destroy the renal parenchyma	Infection by the mycobacterium tuberculosis		urinalysis

WORKSHEET – CLINICAL answers must be reviewed by faculty d/t unknown data

1. Record your patient's vital signs in the box

   [   ]

2. Is the patient's systolic blood pressure within normal limits (WNL)?

3. Calculate your patient's mean arterial pressure (MAP). _____

4. Is the MAP adequate or is it too high or too low? _____

5. What are the concerns if the MAP is too high or too low? _____

6. Calculate your patient's pulse pressure. _____

7. Is your patient's pulse pressure WNL, narrow, or wide? _____

8. What are the normal parameters of pulse pressure? _____

9. What are the normal parameters of a heart rate? _____

10. Is your patient's heart rate too high or too low? _____

11. What are the normal parameters of the respiratory rate? _____

12. What is the concern of tachypnea or bradypnea? (hint- pH level)
    _____.

13. What is the concern of an elevated temperature? _____

14. List reasons the pulse oximetry may not read accurately?
    _____
    _____.

www.ingramcontent.com/pod-product-compliance
Lightning Source LLC
Chambersburg PA
CBHW082243220526
45469CB00009B/2863